NEW WILD ORDER

NEW WILD ORDER

HOW ANSWERING THE CALL OF THE WILD MIGHT JUST SAVE YOUR LIFE (AND SANITY)

ANDY HAMILTON

SCRIBE

Melbourne | London | Minneapolis

Scribe Publications
18–20 Edward St, Brunswick, Victoria 3056, Australia
2 John St, Clerkenwell, London, WC1N 2ES, United Kingdom
3754 Pleasant Ave, Suite 100, Minneapolis, Minnesota 55409, USA

Published by Scribe 2025
Copyright © Andy Hamilton 2025

All rights reserved. Without limiting the rights under copyright reserved above, no part of this publication may be reproduced, stored in or introduced into a retrieval system, or transmitted, in any form or by any means (electronic, mechanical, photocopying, recording or otherwise) without the prior written permission of the publishers of this book.

The moral rights of the author have been asserted.

The advice in this book is not intended to replace the services of trained health professionals or be a substitute for medical advice. You are advised to consult with your health care professional with regard to matters relating to your health, and in particular regarding matters that may require diagnosis or medical attention.

Internal illustrations by Joe McLaren.

Typeset in Portrait by the publishers

Printed and bound in the UK by CPI Group (UK) Ltd,
Croydon CR0 4YY

Scribe is committed to the sustainable use of natural resources and the use of paper products made responsibly from those resources.

978 1 915590 30 5 (hardback)
978 1 761386 07 7 (ebook)

scribepublications.com.au
scribepublications.co.uk
scribepublications.com

*To my sister, Sharon, and my Auntie Christine,
for accepting and encouraging me across a lifetime —
no matter how wild I was — thank you.*

CONTENTS

INTRODUCTION: **The Call of the Wild**   1

CHAPTER ONE: **Life**   21

CHAPTER TWO: **Consciousness**   49

CHAPTER THREE: **Shelter**   89

CHAPTER FOUR: **Bodies**   121

CHAPTER FIVE: **Music**   159

CHAPTER SIX: **Art**   193

CHAPTER SEVEN: **Sleep**   211

CHAPTER EIGHT: **Death**   233

Further Reading   253

Acknowledgements   259

Endnotes   265

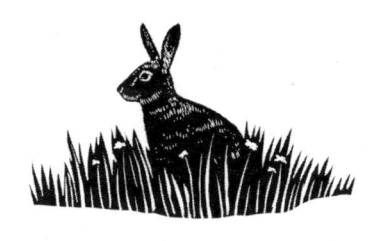

INTRODUCTION

The Call of the Wild

'Tell me and I'll forget; show me and I may remember; involve me and I'll understand.'

CONFUCIUS, 5TH CENTURY

I read the headline: 'Ring of Death'. The accompanying photo had red 'x's marked where people had been murdered in my local town. This was the 1980s, and I was a child only just starting to notice the world outside the bubble I was growing up in, a bubble that wasn't feeling quite as safe as it had when I was very small.

It was a decade that was bookended by the birth of home computers and the subsequent rise of electronic dance music and rave culture; it was also dubbed the decade 'When Violence was the Norm'.[1] Troubles existed worldwide, but youngsters here in the UK were witness to the miners' strike, the Troubles in Northern Ireland, race riots, corporal punishment in school, high unemployment, the AIDS crisis, heroin, Black Wednesday, massive inequalities, and the constant threat of nuclear war. It was a world that felt about as far from a nurturing hotbed of optimism as you could get.

Frustration and anger played out across the country and were, as ever, more acutely felt in poorer areas. Small battles and large battles were seemingly being fought everywhere. The disquiet we felt as a nation was evident in our towns, cities, and villages. I looked at the ring of 'x's, noticing that it circled our house. It was the first time I realised that, even in my town, some people might not live the way I did.

I was one of the lucky ones. I had an alternative world to escape to. The less than salubrious area we lived in meant that my parents could afford a bigger house and a huge garden. And that meant — although, yes, if you strode out of our front door, you found yourself in the middle of a 'ring of death' — if you wandered out of the back door, it was a different story entirely. To a small child, our 50-metre-long garden seemed to stretch out infinitely, into a different world, a world where I could escape some of the realities of the place and time we lived in.

It was there in that suburban back garden that I heard the call of the wild for the first time. I was about seven years old, standing in the dappled shade of our small patch of 70-year-old pine trees.

We'd arrived back from a fortnight's summer holiday under canvas somewhere in the Welsh mountains. My August birthday often coincided with our annual getaway, and I always felt more mature when I returned. The change of light, the temperature, and the first smells of autumn decay marked the turning of the season inside and outside of my being; this signified the end of a chapter in my life, the end of another year.

When we arrived home, I rushed down to the bottom of the garden to check on my base camp, where I noticed a plant growing atop a trench freshly dug the morning before we'd left: the vivid green and tiny white flowers illuminated by the last rays of fading light, stark against the bare mud; a brief gust of wind blowing these small individual plants in the same direction, the uniformity of movement suggesting a single entity, like a branch of tree blowing in a stronger wind. The vision of that plant on that day has stayed with me across my life; I felt powerfully drawn to plants from then on. It wouldn't be until years later that I'd identify this as a fine crop of edible, tasty, and highly nutritious chickweed — one of the most common of all UK plants. Did the plant stir something inside me, something dormant?

The survival side of the army had always intrigued me, not that I wanted to join — I wasn't really the killing type, but I found a strange fascination in the idea that I could join just to learn their survival skills, and perhaps learn how to be tidy to boot. I wonder if it was because I felt quite lonely; although I had friends, and one very close friend, they were shared with my twin brother, who was always a little more charismatic than me, or so I worried. But I never felt lonely in the garden, in the company of nature. I was learning the difference between solitude and loneliness rather early on. It was impossible to feel lonely when you had trees, plants, and squirrels all around.

Down at the bottom of the garden, I could easily forget the world, the playground full of people who'd rather play with each other. I could instead create my own world. In that world, the natural world, there was always something new to find. Beetles to watch running, hoverflies that darted from one place to the next, new plants to look at, and dens to build with my brother. The small patch of grass between the trees felt like part of a great plain, and the tall trunks of the eight pines seemed to scrape the heavens. This felt like a kingdom as large as any country, and more than enough to fill me with a sense of belonging.

I also thought that if I could just survive off my own wits, I would never need to rely on a group; I would be able to live in nature indefinitely, and so I wouldn't be lonely ever again. This feeling, coupled with the chickweed's miraculous appearance that summer, set a compass point that my life would follow: though I did not realise it, I fell in love with edible plants at that very moment.

A month later, I found a recipe in one of my mum's books, for nettle soup. I decided I must make my own; I'm sure I thought it would be the first step towards being able to live off my wits.

Unfortunately, by this time, it was late September, and still too early for the last flush of young nettles before winter. The ones I found were ready to set seed — dark, long, stringy, and rather angry-looking. Although the book clearly said to avoid them or just to gather the top bits, I wanted to follow the weights and measurements in the recipe to the letter. After what seemed like hours searching for younger specimens on my own in the fading light, I looked down into my bag and knew my efforts wouldn't be enough. The garden felt long; longer and lonelier than usual. The sun had already slunk off for its nightly snooze and the final rays of light were reflecting through the apple trees at Number

Two; time was fast running out. Reassuring myself with that fatal thought, 'What's the worst that could happen?', within moments the bag was filled with long, stringy, sorry-looking nettles.

The soup was vile! Nettles that are old are putting their energy into setting seed and they really don't want to be eaten. Some plants will increase their bitterness as they set seed; the nettle, however, defends its next generation with an increase in uric acid, the same acid found in wee. Not only that, but the acid crystallises and the leaves start to develop a sandy texture. My family are not prone to false gratitude, and my soup was duly panned by all.

Somehow undeterred, I continued my quest for wild food and a wild life to go with it.

Inspiration came again a few months later when I saw a man on the local evening news eating flowers. We had my favourite Aunty Christine staying, and I think I also wanted to show off. So, after a few moments of deliberation, I wandered out of the living room and into the dining room. There, on the windowsill, tucked behind gaudy yellow seventies-style curtains, sat a tall brown ceramic vase. Inside the vase, wilting and browning, a forgotten week-old daffodil lingered. Supper, I thought. But this was not a supper that my body wanted to digest, and I can still remember how the yellow contrasted with my blue sleeping bag and brown sofa — we'd given up our bedroom to our auntie — when I saw that daffodil coming right back up again. Here I learned a very valuable lesson — not all flowers are edible!

Joining the Cubs and then the Scouts was the logical, and perhaps the safest, next step towards answering my call of the wild.

My experience in the Scouts starkly contrasted with what I was going through at school. I was the quiet kid; I'd have been called painfully shy back then, but, considering the symptoms of general anxiety disorder,[2] I do wonder if I was suffering from that. It was a painful time: if anyone outside my small friendship group spoke to me, especially a girl, I'd go bright red and fill with panic. I worried about nuclear war. I had tons of time off school due to stomach aches, and almost everything in this violence-scape terrified me. But I was a dichotomy. I'd become good at judo, winning a gold medal for best in the county. All the other boys wanted to challenge me. I was terrified of them, but they kept coming at me. One by one, every break time, I fought the toughest boys in my year. I beat them all without having to throw a punch, but still I lived in a state of abject fear. No one tried to stop this: not my friends, not the teachers or dinner ladies, no one. I felt painfully alone. I think this was my first bout of depression. I was about ten.

This all happened during the winter months, a period when our break times changed: instead of playing in the vast, expansive fields at the back of the school, we were hemmed into the tiny tarmacked playground at the front. Equally, visits to either of the local parks became less frequent, and the garden door stayed shut during these months. With the wisdom of 40 or more years of reflection, I now feel sure that I — and many of the other children I played with — was suffering from nature depletion. An all-too-familiar problem, and one I'll address in the following chapters.

Friendships felt different when we were out in the fields, closer somehow, and during these times loneliness wasn't a problem. That was as long as I played football. I hated football — I was rubbish at most ball sports — but I wanted to be in a group that I contributed to. I'd always play in goal, a position most crappy sportsmen will know. But the practice made me a great goalkeeper; anything was possible in this seemingly wild place.

Having said that, the Scouts offered more time outdoors even in the winter months, and another chance to develop some self-confidence without having to go in goal. As a Scout, I didn't worry about fights, girls, nuclear war, or anything else. It was a revelation that I could now share some of the wild with others, that they too enjoyed a slightly wilder life. Both in goal and in the Scouts I was starting to understand what it was to be part of something in the natural world.

We had access to a woodland campsite that we could use whenever we wanted. Once, we set up camp in February, awaking to a thick blanket of snow on the ground. It felt so calm, natural, and above all comfortable, like I was in my true home. Sure, we might have sneaked a few cans of lager, and occasionally experimented with blowing things up on the fire — we were no angels. But above all, we were there as we had a desire to be outside. Perhaps we all needed that escape. To experience life like it might have been in the simpler times that stretched out behind us. Granted, the past we dreamed about was idealised; erased were the threats of disease, animal and human attacks, and starvation. Still, it felt like we were experiencing a taster of a life that we at least had some control over. A quality of life that feels rare in our society, especially when you are young.

The moments we spent in those woodlands still held the pressures of male hierarchy; there was no getting away from that. We also met Scouts from across the city who came from more salubrious, richer areas, and who could afford to use the tuck shop. But in the woods it felt different; we looked for similarities more often than differences. We aimed to find a way to get on, and our differences didn't seem quite so important. I started to feel like, perhaps, I could live out a nuclear war between the trees. In reality it was still far-fetched, but at least I found some reassurance.

At summer camp, I begged the leaders to teach me to skin a rabbit after finding one dead in a nearby field. I watched, mesmerised, as the brutal but necessary steps were taken and the cute and furry animal became meat. A vegetarian at the time, it was still a skill I never forgot, picking it up again when making a TV pilot in adulthood. We learned how to make shelters cosy enough to sleep inside. I can remember feeling a shift in my being at every Scout camp. It always happened around day three: the colours would change, I'd become happier, and I'd feel closer to the earth around me.

Then, as a very young teen, over one very memorable evening, I discovered the ancient, rhythmic, repetitive drumbeats and the characteristic Roland TB-303 bassline tweaks that characterised the newly emerging music known as acid house — music that seemed to trigger something primal inside me, something joyous. Acid house gave us an excuse to dance like no one was watching, particularly in those early days when the new rules of the dance floor were being formed. Gone were the stylised moves of Michael Jackson, the slow dances to ballads, and the hard head-banging of heavy metal. The dance floor was somewhere I could feel the comfort of connection in a place other than my garden; instead of being alone, I was part of something bigger — I felt the unity of a dance floor. When I reflect on the power that music had, I can't help feeling that I had found the modern equivalent of the psychoacoustic, or brain-altering, sound of the shamanic drum. These were sounds I couldn't ignore, beats that the whole adult world called dangerous: the *devil's music*. Newspaper headlines warned of the perils of this music alongside the dangers of Ecstasy, or 'E', the party drug that often accompanied it. I desperately wanted in.

I was totally sober that first night I found acid house, but I remember letting people think I was on drugs — it was easier than to admit the fact that I was just having fun. That I loved to dance with no holds barred.

The truth, though, was that I was also drawn to drink and drugs; I craved them. Even at the time, I couldn't quite work out why. Carl Jung might say that this was because addiction could temporarily alleviate the anxieties I was feeling.[3] That, for a blissful moment, I could forget about being shy, nuclear war, and why I found French so difficult. I didn't have to think about the lad, neglected by his alcoholic and abusive parents, who wanted to take out his frustrations on me every morning on the way into school. We were the *posh* kids, with our slightly bigger house with a huge garden, after all. His street fighting, complete with sticks and random bits of metal, was more than a match for my judo. It was also because I felt these lifestyle choices appeared cool. I could stand out as rebellious and be accepted. I could forge an identity separate from my twin brother. Conversely, the Scouts felt uncool, and soon I'd be kicked out, giving me the excuse I needed to be rid of it despite perhaps still needing it and still enjoying it. As we all know, sometimes teenagers can be their own worst enemies.

I still spent a lot of time outdoors, but back then that meant hanging around outside the youth club smoking dope (cannabis). Or sitting outside shops drinking as much booze as we could get our hands on. Maybe Jung was right, as something ate away inside me. People talked about moderation — richer, less frustrated kids, mostly — but I couldn't get enough. Trouble is, once you are in that lifestyle of excess, it can take hold, and little did I know that it was the start of a cycle that would last for around 20 years or more.

By the time I was 15, I was smoking two packs of Marlboro a day, regularly smoking cannabis, and drinking whenever I could either afford it or someone else had some to share. I'd also started taking LSD. You have to remember there was a culture of this at the time; drinking almost felt like something to aspire to, something cool, and being able to drink more than others or take more drugs gave you kudos — we were all a bit broken.

No one really talked about mental health, and the world felt hopeless and violent. I can remember someone older, an ex-hippy, chastising us that while his generation took drugs to expand their minds, we took them to close ours. Maybe we just had stuff to shut out.

Yet, the fact that much of this happened outdoors in all weathers and within a group of friends is reassuring. I hadn't fallen too far away from the core that made me who I still am today. I was obviously dealing with something, but despite the excess — maybe because of it — it was a happy time. I'd done away with school-related anxieties by simply not going, sitting about in the woods or walking the fields around the school instead. I found this was more nurturing, and a far more fun environment than a 1980s school, with all its archaic teaching practices and overworked teachers who themselves didn't always turn up.

Before I turned 16, I left what little schooling I'd had behind and started working full-time in an apprenticeship that was to set me up for life. Snobbish peer pressure from judgemental friends urging me to leave, depression, drug use, and a workplace that, as many places did back then, hummed with the threat of toxic masculinity meant I lasted only a few months. My anxiety spiralled out of control, and I'd reached a crisis point. I returned to education, joining a college with a little woodland and a park opposite. I met new and exciting friends, including Doug, a very sweet and creative fella, who had dropped out of private school for similar reasons to why I had left my apprenticeship.

Doug introduced me to Cornwall, and the simple pleasure of feeling sand beneath my feet and all the pressures of teenage life ebbing away. It seems odd to recall that we only spent two weekends there, considering the influence it had. We were living off Pot Noodles and baked beans, and we didn't do anything special: we'd meet up and hang out with many of his friends or his dad, swim, paddle, and simply have fun. People loved him there; he'd been coming since he was a child, and it felt like it was his playground, a place where he really belonged. A place that felt wild. I wanted to go there again and again.

Tragically, Doug died soon after we met, but the memory of the place and our time in Cornwall had a transformative effect. Soon after his death, I rather disastrously tried to move down there for life, this time lasting two months.

Although, the move wasn't a complete failure, as it led to an enlightened experience, an accidental stumbling into a forgotten archaic practice that would give me strength in the dark moments that were to follow. A practice which, I now think, if done correctly, could benefit much of our youth. Something that I'll explore later in this book.

But for now, Doug's death simply left a deep hole inside me. We had connected as true friends, and I needed that connection with others, though I did not always know how to come by it.

Through dance music, again, I found a group of talented misfits like myself, who rejoiced in moving to each and every thumping sound, from the kick drum to the tom-tom and the snare, until the summer's morning sun beat against our faces and our dance-weary bodies begged us to stop. We'd fill ourselves with substances that opened our hearts to each other and connected us with the divine — at least, that's what I told myself, though perhaps I just wanted to be off my face, to momentarily forget about my grief for my friend.

One morning, full of Ecstasy and mushrooms, I could hear something in the distance. A drumming? Or something else? I wondered if it was an audio hallucination until I felt the noise coming closer: it was a hoof-hit rhythm beaten by wild horses. The morning mist hung above the nearby river, and the horses appeared through it. Majestic, vibrant, and alive. The noise got louder and louder until it seemed to vibrate and trigger the ancient inside me. I'd regale friends at the pub with events like this, or the fact that I enjoyed a sunset or a walk in the park, never putting them together to realise that I loved these things so much because I was getting some kind of nature therapy. That term wouldn't make it to my little bubble of existence for another 20 years.

It was easier back then to just take off for a weekend and do things like this. Rents (when they were actually paid) were low, bills could mostly be ignored, and credit was available. Few of us had any responsibilities, expectations were low, and hedonism ruled.

Those times soon changed, though, and we all went our separate ways, finding jobs we could stick to, starting families, and becoming adults. The *civilised* world trapped me. For a while I was in and out of low-paying jobs, doing everything from packing clothes in a warehouse, to sorting post, throwing massive slabs of meat into a machine, and inputting data. None of these jobs were what you would call fulfilling. I'd moved out of my parents' house with its big back garden and into the maze of Victorian terraces nearer town. Everything felt grey and lifeless, and something inside me was slowly dying.

Closer to town, and the threat of street violence had increased. My age didn't help; assaults by young men on young men are the most common, after all.[4] I had a few minor beatings and witnessed some more major ones, narrowly missed getting a razor blade across my cheek, and just got away from an iron bar round the back of my skull after being chased by 20 or more young men and remaining helpless as my brother felt the full force. Consequently, I started to drink more frequently, and it became my main pastime. This, of course, meant I ended up in insecure housing, once forcibly evicted: pulled by my hair down the stairs, kicked in the face, and thrown onto the street. Not everyone appreciates living with a drinker and the chaos that can bring. I shifted in and out of depression. I did not yet know, or perhaps just could not remember, how to release myself from that spiral.

Thoughts of wild food and wild living lay dormant over these years, until I moved away from the built-up, back-to-back housing of a city that was then failing and into a city where you could see greenery almost anywhere. I met Emma, whose love helped me believe in myself again. Together, we got an allotment, started going on long walks in the countryside, and cooked fresh produce, making drinks like elderflower champagne. My brother had an allotment, too, and we spoke about starting a website. I struck while the iron was hot, downloaded a bunch of pirated software, and taught myself just enough coding to create something that looked a little different from what everyone else was doing. In those early days, there were more journalists using the net than there were people actually putting stuff up. And we were doing something a little different, so of course we attracted the attention of the media and launched our careers.

With the space to experiment and be who I wanted to be, I flourished. I bought a copy of Richard Mabey's *Food for Free*, and I was like a caged animal released. I memorised every plant in that book, tried out every suggestion of how to cook them. At that time, there were scant books on wild food, but I tracked down and read them all. Emma and I hadn't been together long. Every walk we went on had me crouching down to take a photo or scribbling down stages of plant growth in a notebook. She tells me now that the notes weren't too bad, but taking endless photos of plants was rather boring. Indeed, some people have tons of photos of their shared experiences before kids came along — I've got thousands of photos of plants, trees, and fungi. Lucky Emma.

It was all good experience, a good background to start a career with plants. I can remember having a target: I wanted to be able to look out of a train window at the plants that grew between the tracks and be able to identify them all. When I could do this whenever a train stopped, I'd know I'd reached that target. It came soon enough, and I started to teach foraging, learning much from my students. Over time, I learned enough about wild food to be able to forage myself a meal wherever I was in the UK. I could roast a dandelion, thistle or burdock root, tiptoe along a seashore for seaweeds and molluscs, and sift through a wild patch of garden for edible salad crops.

Hard drugs became a distant memory; I didn't need the escape quite as much anymore. I had found a route to happiness in the wild, and I had a woman who loved me, even in my darkest moments. Moments that came less frequently. A natural humanity was starting to weave its way back in. I was finding my New Wild Order.

I quit my now 60-a-day smoking habit, cut down on drinking (despite having discovered the alchemy of home brewing), and kept foraging. I was living the good life. However, though I was writing about foraging, gardening, brewing my own beer, and being outdoors, I found myself increasingly sat in front of a computer, administering what was supposed to be success but felt like burnout.

Having worked in jobs that I'd hated for so long, now that I had somehow managed to start writing and foraging for a living, how could I let this go? Believing that days in front of a computer were where the real work was, I was getting addicted to that world. I ran a web forum; it was a nurturing and supportive environment, and many people who visited became real-life friends. But I can't deny a darker side; that I didn't also feel something of the same hit that glues many people to their smartphones and social media today. I was replacing the hit of one addiction with another.

It was a slow and steady process to pull myself away from my screen, from the grip of the digital prison and the comfortable cage of civilisation that many of us find ourselves incarcerated inside. I mean, don't get me wrong, I like going to the cinema, drinking in pubs, hopping on a bus, and hot showers. But I find peace in the natural world. I always have.

Luckily, the wild always knows when to call me back. And it did again now. I soon found myself plucking and eating raw oysters from the shores of Scottish islands, eating pollock, feasting on urchins and scallops fresh from the sea floor. I made tea with psychotropic plants until I could feel what it was to be part of a forest. One year, I consumed the plants in just one valley — so that my bones and body were as much a part of that place as the leaves on the trees. Holidays got wilder, too, and I found a taste for wild water flowing from hillsides and learned where it was safe to drink. I was sharing this world with Emma whenever I could. We climbed mountains, followed badger tracks until they became barbed-wire fences, and crossed waterfalls, our boots rarely staying mud-free. She stayed by my side, and helped me realise I could achieve more than just being the last in the pub. I wasn't always getting the balance of work and wild right — money is an issue, after all. But I was making big tracks in that direction.

How my experiences of violence relate to yours will vary, from shocking to all too familiar. Yet, many of us have some kind of crap in our lives that we'd like to deal with. Many of us have demons to face, and the wild world is out there to make this job easier.

The process described in the following pages profoundly changed me, helping to release me from past mistakes. You may feel that some of my experiences are inaccessible, of another time and place — but they are of the here and now. Even if you read this in the far-off future, they are of a now that (I hope) you'll still be able to access.

I hope to help you answer your own call of the wild by teaching you skills that would allow you to escape some of the ills of our society. To take you by the hand and reveal the wild spots that I'm certain will be near to your home, no matter how small they might be. Places that would lower your stress and anxiety levels, and where we could find plants to fill our bellies, all with very little effort. Indeed, I live between two major roads, in a house on a 1960s housing estate. I do the school run every day, and have professional and personal responsibilities, financial and familial commitments; in other words, I have just as many obligations and responsibilities as the next person. In this last year, I have become an unpaid carer for a family member suffering with chronic fatigue/long Covid, a stressful and upsetting experience. Yet, because of my past experiences, I know that I can find solace in nature and wild living, so this was also the year I embraced joy, the year I felt more alive than I ever have before, the year I reminded myself how much the world around me has to offer. It was the year that

I started to get the balance right at a time when I needed it the most, learning the value in contemplation and that healing the past is endlessly more productive than repeating it.

The New Wild Order that I try to live my life by now isn't really anything new: it's a way of being that has always been available to us, if only we could embrace it. You might think you need to travel to remote places to experience wild living, but you don't. Most of what I speak of in this introduction, and between now and the back cover of this book, happened inside my country, much of it no more than 50 miles (80 kilometres) from the front door of my house in Bristol or my hometown of Northampton — both of them fairly typical urban landscapes.

Nor do these experiences need a huge amount of knowledge. The pages that follow aren't about aspirational living; they are about practical living. They are about looking at the world around you and finding where it's at fault, rather than blaming yourself. This book is about a way of life that is more in tune with how humans should feel and interact with each other and the world around us, and about dropping the comfortable prison we continue to create for ourselves to find the real freedom and happiness we all deserve.

I invite you to embrace the New Wild Order with me. To start seeing the world for how it really is, to experience its beauty, and to flourish as a human. To breathe air made by plants and trees rather than air conditioners, to feel the warmth and light from the sun rather than heaters and light bulbs, to not just see beauty and wonder through a screen, but to see it and, more importantly, feel it with all your senses. And I invite you to connect with our fellow humans in forgiving and nurturing ways that unite rather than divide.

Let's take one step at a time, and maybe you too will start to wonder if it's your comfort zone that is making you uncomfortable. And maybe, like me, you'll find what sanity looks like in an insane world.

CHAPTER ONE

Life

'All good things are wild and free.'
HENRY DAVID THOREAU, 1863

There is an old adage that suggests that if you fall in love with your job, you'll never do a day's work again. As I write — usually about foraging — I've a broad smile across my face. I'm looking out of the window at the yellowing leaves of my hop bine and apple trees swaying in the increasingly strong November winds. A small flock of goldfinches, *Carduelis carduelis* L., characteristically bounce across the stark white cloud cover. Their number has barely dwindled since the summer, a sure sign that our hedgerow is now an established part of the local environment. The abundance of what many would call weeds, and the firethorn, *Pyracantha* L., which has grown so much that most of it occupies our tolerant neighbours' garden, offers them plenty of food during the winter.

Goldfinches are part migratory. This means that some of them will fly off to Spain when food is scarce. Others choose to stay if they think they can survive. The fact that the winter flock is bigger than last year is a reassuring sign that our efforts to help the local wildlife are working.

Just like the goldfinches, I'm content with where I sit, and, like them, I feel reassured in the knowledge that I can see food sources around me. Walnut and hazelnut trees, and, in a pinch, even the squirrels that frequent them. Apples, blackberries, red and blackcurrants, gooseberries, strawberries, rosehips, hawthorn, bullace, tayberry, dandelion, nettle, and alexanders all grow in my garden, just a two-mile walk from central Bristol. I can step outside and gather a highly nutritious meal in less than a few minutes.

This feels natural, the basis of what is right in my New Wild Order. I feel led by my own intuition rather than what is available as a two-for-one offer. Food is crucial for our existence and it seems a good place to start in my quest.

Although we like to forget it, we are no different than the goldfinches, and we have to ensure we live in a place that can sustain us. Even in an urban environment, I often forage a partly wild diet, picking a few things at a time to supplement food from the organic veg box we get every Friday. When I'm returning home after dropping the kids off at school, I might pluck off a few nettle seeds, or munch on a dandelion or sow thistle leaf. If I'm lucky, I might find a hazelnut that I'll crack between rocks. On longer trips, I fill carrier bags full of wild produce which I then process for storage: drying mushrooms, freezing mixed-leaf hummus, or fermenting wild garlic seeds.

It's a far cry from a flat I used to share in Nottingham. A place with no living or dining room, a tiny kitchen, thin floors, and a lethal set of wooden stairs that in dry weather took you up to the front door — in the rain they became a slide. I had access to food there, as the flat was situated above a shop that sold bacon rolls. The smell came up through the gaps in the floorboards every morning. I was in hideous debt, had no education, and couldn't hold down a job. If I'd had the knowledge then that I have now, I would have been able to walk down the streets to a local park where I could make up a plate of nutritious plants; back then, I couldn't always afford even a cheap, greasy white roll from the shop downstairs. The smell was a constant reminder that I was unable to sustain myself.

Alas, it's a situation that many can relate to, and it will hopefully seem odd to future generations that many of us here in the UK are currently reliant on food banks. Of the 6.2 million people on Universal Credit,[1] over half (according to the hunger charity The Trussell Trust)[2] report that they have had to resort to using a food bank in the last month. That's 3.4 million people, or 5 per cent of the country, in the fifth richest country in the world.[3] These are people who find themselves in a similar situation to mine back then, or much worse.

It's true that a wild diet might go some way to alleviating that. However, things would have to change. Although education about wild food is changing and we now see far more people gathering food than ever before, it's not reached the point that it's become commonplace. I know, too, that in some cultures foraging can even be looked down on; the unharvested wild fruit in Amhara, Ethiopia, is testament to that.[4] Indeed, it was like that here about fifteen years ago, and I had a stand-up row with someone who was certain I shouldn't be harvesting fruit from trees. She was sure it was poisonous. Even now, people will give me funny looks as I harvest food from urban areas.

There is also the issue of land use and how everything from our language to our law favours its destruction. The word 'wasteland' is absent from these pages and from my last foraging book. It used to mean land that isn't *put to work* to farm crops nor for buildings. Therefore, a heath, a forest, and a beach are all wastelands, as indeed is land that is reverting back to its wild state. Land that is often full of wild plants which can eaten. This land is often sold to *developers* — who'll ensure that it can be turned into something useful.* Maybe an office block, a car park, a road, or a Pot Noodle factory.

Lastly, in order to forage sustainably, I personally think that there needs to be agency to farm wild foods. That might seem like an oxymoron — after all, food can only be farmed *or* wild. Yet, evidence is emerging to suggest that this might be exactly how we have sustainably lived in our landscape for as long as we have. As long ago as almost 11,600 BC, we could have been manipulating the land around us, as José Iriarte at the University of Exeter suggests.[5] Littered around the savannahs of Bolivia, curious but fertile mounds have been found — 6,000 of them, all about one hectare in size. It is thought that compost made from human waste enriched

---

* Even the word 'developer' favours the developers; it's a word that itself *developed* in the 18th century and means 'bring out the potential in'. Although, and perhaps ironically, the word potentially derives from a Middle English word meaning 'caustic medicine'.

the soil, which was then used to grow Brazil nut trees, squash, cassava, and peach trees.

It's important to note that these were not farmers; they were more like wild gardeners. That they were cultivating plants which were already there, enriching the environment and not planting mono-crops, degrading the soil, and using unsustainable farming practices.[6] Manipulating the environment might seem like it is going against something wild, yet beavers, ants, and elephants all do this, too. It's not about changing the environment, but how you change it.

In my garden, for example, I've planted the fruit bushes and fruit trees, but the walnut arrived via a squirrel — wild. There are other plants there, too, such as the dandelions, nettles, and sow thistles that have all grown here without the need for cultivation. These all add to the reassurance that, if I needed to, I could live on wild food alone. It's also nice to be able to share this with my children and their friends, who love the idea of living in the wild, too, as with that comes a freedom — one that we, as a species, have sadly lost. I know that if I ever found myself in the same situation that I did 25 years ago in Nottingham, I wouldn't have to rely on earning a living to feed my family — though, granted, there would be a bit of resistance to get my kids to eat a fully wild diet!

Yet, the wild diet might also offer another freedom: one from crop failure caused by climate change. This is a point of view put forward by Adrian Jaeggi, a professor at the University of Zurich's Institute of Evolutionary Medicine. Jaeggi says that when people live in a climate that is unpredictable, the nomadic hunting-and-gathering lifestyle is favourable compared to farming.[7] The boom of farming happened between 11,000 and 10,000 years ago; before then, when humans predominantly lived as hunter-gatherers, the climate was all over the place, colder and prone to peaks and troughs.

As we enter a time of massive climate change, it seems obvious that we should be considering alternative ways of living and eating. Almost half the world relies on getting most of its calorific intake from just one species of plant — grass. More specifically, cereal crops (the types of grass that are grown to be eaten) make up a massive 45 per cent of our present diet.[8] And that's before we consider the 4 billion hectares of grain that are eaten indirectly in the form of animal feed.[9] The future of food is rather precarious, and it's a little terrifying.

I do find some reassurance in knowing how much we could diversify our diets if we needed to, though. We might mostly eat just a small handful of crops now, yet almost anything with a calorific value can be found on the menu in some corner of the world. Foods that are rejected by some cultures are devoured and savoured by others. I've sat around tables serving puffer fish, fish lips, monkey brains, fried spiders, ducks' feet, ants, crickets, eyeballs, frogs' legs, overfed goose liver, and grilled sheep's head. Some of these foods I tried, some I may never eat. Equally, some of you reading or listening to this would never eat foods that I love, like blue cheese, fermented squirrel tongue, or perhaps the most heinous: Pot Noodle.

Our dietary preferences are driven by a number of factors, such as culture, socioeconomic status, and disease diagnoses,[10] as well as genes. Culture is perhaps the biggest influence. I've only seen insects on the menu once, and it was here in Bristol. They were served to me as an appetiser in a Mexican restaurant that has since closed down, yet they are eaten in 80 per cent of the countries on this planet.[11] High up in the Arctic Circle, you'll find a diet of 95 per cent meat favoured by many of the Inuit people; over in India, you can find the opposite, as up 39 per cent of the population (or 563 million people) is vegetarian. These diets are examples of how the landscape can affect what we eat. Although climate change is having a significant impact, the Arctic is, for now, still a barren landscape; even in the summer, temperatures rarely reach above 10°C (50°F). For most of the year, this means it is covered in snow and therefore devoid of green, with soil so solid that you'd need a pneumatic drill just to plant a seed — a seed that would have little hope of germinating. In contrast, India has monsoon for four months of the year, and temperatures that, in some places, reach in the mid-40s Celsius (over 100°F). These hot and humid conditions increase the risk of meat becoming contaminated and going rotten, making a vegetarian diet not just a religious choice but a wise one.

Another wise food choice might be seaweed, especially for those living on islands. Over in Japan, seaweed is eaten more than anywhere else in the world, and they have one of the highest life expectancies on the planet.[12] This could suggest that seaweeds could be a crucial part of a healthier diet; seaweed does, after all, contain high-quality protein boasting all nine essential amino acids.

Consider that seaweed needs no pesticides, fertilisers, herbicides or ploughing, and current farming methods mean that seaweed is also much cheaper and more sustainable to grow than conventional vegetables. It has been called an underwater forest; just as a terrestrial forest does, it can absorb carbon and purify its surroundings. If that wasn't enough to convince you of its virtues, a seaweed farm offers a further benefit to marine life, often restoring habitats for sea otters, fish, and urchins.

There is little doubt that our pre-agriculture ancestors lived a more sustainable life than us, but did they eat seaweed? According to eminent professor and archaeologist Jon M Erlandson, they certainly did at one point. In his 2007 and subsequent 2018 papers,[13,14] Erlandson hypothesises that a nutrient-rich kelp highway joined Japan with Alaska approximately 16,000 years ago. A bountiful feast for seafarers travelling down from Asia, via Australia, and over to the Americas. Erlandson argues that it was this highway that enabled our species, *Homo sapiens*, to spread out across the Americas — not a land bridge, as has been claimed previously. The land bridge theory suggests we dispersed around the globe across straits that surfaced as sea levels fell during the Ice Age. From the point of view of a forager, I find this hard to believe: there are some edible plants that grow worldwide, but many of these only spread much more recently, during colonisation, so how would the travellers have known what was safe to eat on the long crossing?

Like humans, plants and animals have evolved very differently according to their varied habitats and conditions, and therefore there is a huge difference between what you'll find in one region and the next. Locked in by geographical details, sometimes land species may be specific to just one region. Changes in soil types, shade (or lack of), and availability of water will all furnish an area with different plants. Just take the plants found across the land mass of the United States, for example, which outside the vast expanse of China has the most diverse range of temperate floras in the world. The native plants differ beyond recognition from one side of the country to the other: you couldn't grow a pecan tree in upstate New York, and a red chokeberry bush would struggle in the arid conditions of Texas.

On land, one could die or be seriously injured from eating plants like hemlock, which might look very much like very edible plants in the wild carrot family, such as wild carrot, parsnip, and sweet cicely, but which contain a lethal poison. Mistaking one plant for another, especially if your calorie intake was low, could be disastrous — fatal, even.

Japan and America are terrestrially very different, and yet the ocean between them is one. Even children would have had no trouble identifying seaweeds, mammals, and sea birds along the kelp highway; they would have been just the same as those at home.

With oysters, mussels, sea lions, whale, seaweed, and much more on the menu every night, seafaring migrants would have been a very healthy bunch, getting all the nutrients and benefits a coastal diet affords. In contrast, if these early humans had migrated across land routes, they would have been in a sorry state; most, if not all, would not have made it across vast areas of land that have little or no, or only unfamiliar, food. They also would have encountered many obstacles, and changing temperatures would have meant massive ice melt, causing rapidly flowing rivers that would have been impossible to cross.

In a cave known as Hoyo Negro (Black Hole) on Mexico's Yucatán, paleoscientists found the remains of a 15- or 16-year-old girl, standing just 1.5 metres (4 feet 10 inches) tall. She is thought to have died around 13,000 years ago.[15]

DNA extracted from her wisdom teeth indicates that she originated from Asia, and it has been suggested that many Native Americans could trace their ancestry back to her. Given the arguments against land-based migration, could her presence in the cave be due to migration across the kelp highway?

The truth is that we don't know. Besides, these sorts of arguments are rarely that clean-cut. Perhaps ancient humans had the seemingly unique capablity of walking and jumping in a boat? Just a thought. I wonder if this played out like many of our family holidays, with me suggesting that we go on some epic long hike and Emma suggesting a day at the beach. Sometimes, just because something is the easier option doesn't mean that everyone took it.

Even so, there is more evidence of human habitation in South America that further supports the idea that ancient humans were seaweed-eaters and probably sailors, too. In a peat bog at Monte Verde, around 500 miles (800 kilometres) south of Santiago, artefacts have been found that are thought to be approximately 14,000 years old, with some reports suggesting an even earlier date of 30,000 years.[16] Between those dates, we were in the middle of a glacial period, an ice age, during which time much of the Earth's water would have been locked up in sea ice, and sea levels would have been much higher. This site would have been some 50 miles (80 kilometres) from the coast, but still the findings included traces of at least 19 species of marine algae. Even in a direct line, this distance takes around a day or two to walk, and about the same amount of time in a canoe, therefore indicating that these particular seaweeds were a very important resource. Not all of the seaweeds found would have been in season all year round, suggesting that they were even important enough to have preserved.

The seaweed was dried. It wasn't just random species of seaweed, and many of the specimens were mixed with other plants. The seaweeds would have been carefully chosen by the inhabitants of Monte Verde for their medicinal and edible qualities; many of the species found are still in use today, both for dietary and medicinal reasons. The findings at Monte Verde and other sites indicate that seaweed was a very important plant for these people; perhaps it has always been that way.

The site in Monte Verde is an intriguing one, as it also sheds some light on just how sophisticated our ancestors were. Two buildings were unearthed. The main one was an 18-metre (60-foot) tent or hut-like structure that could have housed around 30 people. This hut was complete with foundations, floors, and a hearth with cooking facilities, and the whole structure could have even been separated into rooms. The tools that were found on the site included beautifully carved blades, hand axes, and scrapers. The other hut was a little smaller, but complete with a hearth, too. Archaeologists suggest that the smaller structure was a residential area and the other could have been some kind of healthcare facility.

As well as archaeological, there is also evolutionary evidence of our affinity with the sea. Next time you go swimming, or spend too long luxuriously languishing in the bath, have a look at your fingertips, perhaps even your toes. They will have wrinkled up, but have you ever questioned why? Try grabbing wet objects underwater first with unwrinkled fingers, then with wrinkled fingers — your grip should improve when your fingers are wrinkled.[17] The smart money suggests that this is to improve your grip when foraging for seaweed and shellfish.[18] This is because the wrinkles channel water away from your fingers or feet. It's kind of how a bike tyre works. I feel a decreased sensitivity in my fingers when in this state, which is perhaps why we don't have permanently wrinkled fingers.

The case feels watertight for seaweed and seafood to have been integral to the survival of our species. Could seaweed be an important food for our future, too? Considering the problems facing conventional farming, such as soil degradation and climate changes,[19,20] the need for a more diverse food future is now becoming urgent.[21] Bren Smith, a farmer from Stony Creek, Connecticut, believes seaweed could be part of this future. He and his not-for-profit organisation, Greenwave,[22] believe that seaweed farming could be part of a restorative farming future. Indeed, seaweed farming could be the magic bullet that saves us from ourselves, reducing carbon emissions, mitigating ocean acidification, and providing a renewable and clean bio-fuel, whilst offering a home for thousands of marine species.[23]

One thing that I've noticed with coastal foraging is just how easy it is to get a meal and how enjoyable. Good friend and fellow forager Mark Williams describes the intertidal zone and the marshy swamp area that would have surrounded it as prime real estate, in every age before the Mesolithic. Mark is part of a growing wave of people who have re-found the value of our coastlines. His sold-out coastal foraging walks attract international attention; Michelin-starred chefs flock to a dreich* part of west Scotland, paying high prices in order to rediscover this ancient food.

I now always have some foraged seaweed in the kitchen. I use it little and often, adding smoked and dried kelp to a myriad of dishes for flavouring. A little goes a long way: one 10-centimetre (3-inch) strand along with a little dried fish left in 500 millilitres (one pint) of water overnight in the fridge is enough to create some dashi,[24] or if I'm cooking for a vegetarian I switch the fish for mushroom powder. Dashi is a Japanese-style stock that can be used for making soups and broths. I also use pepper dulse — *Osmundea pinnatifida* — as a seasoning, and I harvest laver to make sushi and to snack on.[25] Seaweed might not replace all vegetables in my diet, but it is an important addition.

Foraging may not be the panacea that will cure the world in a future that will most certainly see food shortages, but it is reassuring knowing it could at least help. The idea of a diet that could be positive not just for the environment but also for our health is very appealing, and don't worry, it includes more than just seaweed! Over the last four years I've replaced over 90 per cent of the meat in my diet with wild meat. It is a way of eating meat that isn't as inherently cruel to animals as the process of factory farming.[26] Roadkill would be another consideration if it were more readily available; it's not quite so common near the centre of Bristol — often what could have been eaten is too damaged by traffic. Besides, I'm not entirely sure what the vegetarians

---

* Scottish English meaning continuously grey, damp, and drizzly weather.

in my house would make of me bringing home a badger or a fox to butcher. Considering that 194 million birds and 29 million animals die on European roadsides every year,[27] perhaps it is something I should consider trying on the rare occasions I have the house to myself!

Instead, I have found another way of obtaining meat that would normally go to waste. The current deer cull means that a lot of gourmet meat is ending up in dog bowls or, worse, rubbish bins.[28] The deer population in the UK is currently the highest it's been for 1,000 years, and the cull is an attempt to bring the population down to more manageable proportions. Their high number means deer are starting to cause untold damage to woodlands: eating newly planted trees and hampering natural regeneration.[29] They can also be a hazard to drivers. But perhaps most tragically, high numbers cause damage to the deer themselves. Too many deer and not enough food means a malnourished herd. Eating venison at this moment in time can be seen as a positive act not just for the deer but for the wider environment.

In a land where many of the natural predators have been eradicated, maybe we should be looking at ourselves as a possible positive keystone species, a species that has a large effect on the environment. The native red squirrel, *Sciurus vulgaris*, remains threatened here in the UK, and there are a number of reasons for its decline, including the fact that we have destroyed much of its habitat. Then, to make matters worse, we introduced the invasive grey squirrel, *Sciurus carolinensis*. The greys carry parapoxvirus, a disease that often kills the reds while not appearing to affect the health of the greys. The greys also eat unripe green acorns, while the reds like their acorns ripe. Thus, the greys rid both the red squirrels and us of a valuable food source. If the nutty-tasting greys started to be seen on menus, it could help to control the population. This would be beneficial to our environment: both squirrels eat bird eggs, but the greys will eat as many as 10 times more than the reds. Greys' guts contain oxalate-degrading bacteria,[30] which means they can digest tree bark from oak, beech, hornbeam, and wild cherry, causing tree damage.

I've never taken the life of an animal; I have skinned a few and learned a bit of butchery. As a meat-eater, I feel that it is important I learn these skills. I also think it's important that, one day, I do take the life of an animal for food — especially if it is to help the wider good of the herd and the environment. If you eat meat, maybe it's important to you, too? To know what it feels like to take a life and to do it with reverence for the animal.

Recently, I found myself preparing some game meat for a big feast. As I did, I said a short thank-you to each pheasant I plucked. It felt right and natural. Since then, it's felt a little odd doing the same for the slabs of venison I buy off the internet, but it still feels like the right thing to do; it's become a little silent ritual of mine. Considering that I know how to forage for food, I also think it's important that I don't just rely on someone else to harvest the meat I eat.

But could I actually go through with it, and would I be more comfortable with a vegetarian diet if I did have to kill? A friend of mine, Dan Westall, came face to face with this dilemma. He, his wife, and a few friends appeared in a British TV show on Channel 4 called *Surviving the Stone Age*.[31] To survive, the group had to hunt game. Instead of all going out with bows and arrows, they worked out who was the most capable of hitting a moving target. It is far more beneficial for the flavour of the meat and less cruel to the animal to get a clean kill. It turned out that Dan was head and shoulders the best in the group. But Dan didn't want to be the one to kill an animal, he's a thoughtful and caring chap who's empathy goes beyond thinking of his fellow humans. Killing therefore, had never been on his agenda; yet as a meat eater he knew he was ignoring a universal truth that all of us meat eaters have to face at some point. In order to eat meat, someone has to kill it first.

It was interesting to watch Dan work though his dilemma. Eventually, he did manage to bring down a deer and it helped to feed the group. He felt that eating the deer was the best way to honour its life. It was also very clear that Dan's success meant a much happier group, as they were starting to go hungry. I can quite understand a reluctance to eat meat — I was vegetarian myself for around four years. However, I think it a far bigger crime to let the meat from these magnificent beasts go to waste in a country that has food banks than it is to eat their meat.

It's not just obvious food sources that are going to waste; it's the less obvious, too. Every year, millions of plants that could be used as food are sprayed, pulled out of the ground or burned out of existence. The leading weedkiller in this country, Roundup, has one of them — a dandelion — as a poster child for its products. Its TV adverts state that 'the only good weed is a weed that's dead',[32] further conditioning us to the idea of perfectly bland, perfectly lifeless lawns, instead of areas brimming with food.

Wild food is all around us. I forage it and have done for

years; on occasion, I've even tested the limits and tried to eat a wild-food-only diet. In fact, for lunch today I went out to my garden and pulled up a few alexander (*Smyrnium olusatrum*) roots along with some dandelion roots. I then harvested a few dandelion leaves, a sprig or two of ivy-leaved toadflax (*Cymbalaria muralis*), some nettles (*Urtica dioica*), some plantain (*Plantago major*), and a few walnuts (*Juglans regia*). I roasted the roots, blanched the leaves, and toasted the nuts — sprinkling them on to the leaves. I then topped it all with venison steak that had been marinating in a mixture of nettle miso with alexander pepper and elderberry liqueur. It was delicious, and the gathering took barely any time.

The garden has taken a while to get to this point, and I'd like to introduce more wild plants to make the job of foraging in it easier. I did have a setback a few years ago. My dad was visiting and disappeared to go off and do something useful. He's often found stacking a dishwasher — like me, he likes to grab some moments to himself, and if this is in the service of another, even better. So when he came back in from the garden with a big grin and told me how he'd weeded half of it, I thanked him through gritted teeth.

My dad likes order; his garden (the garden I grew up playing in) is always *almost there* rather than something that can just be enjoyed in all its wild glory. Flower beds get weeded, holly trees (for some reason I'm yet to fathom) get pruned down to next to nothing, as do *weed trees* like elderflower. However, the wild world will often find a way, and I'm pleased to say that not only is the nettle patch I first foraged from still in the same place, so is the first patch of chickweed I found, along with all but one of the pine trees and an ever-increasing patch of brambles. The survival of this little wild Eden is assured, as it's about as far you can get from the house without finding yourself on someone else's property.

Still, foraging is much easier when I get to spend a weekend on a beach.[33] I've made meals using parasol mushrooms from sandy shores, or fresh mussels plucked off the rocks and cooked over hot stones, eaten raw oysters from the shore, caught pollock and eaten it as sushi moments after it was lifted from the sea; I've crisped up wire weed and had it with noodles, slow-cooked limpets in Chardonnay, and eaten fresh sea urchins — all these foods are nutritious and made flavourful meals. Each was gathered in a very short amount of time and eaten as fresh as the day.

However, I don't live near a beach, I live in the city, and so foraging has become something that supplements my diet rather than sustains it fully. Maybe it will be the same for you? I've always wondered, though, if I didn't have to earn money and could devote my time to foraging, could I go longer on a wild-food-only diet, and would it be possible without seafood playing a major role? Luckily, I'm in a unique position to find out, as I have countless friends who experiment with wild food every day.

In the spring of 2023, 24 of them went between one and three months living on a wild-food-only diet for a study conducted by Scottish forager, author, and herbalist — and my friend — Monica Wilde. The rules were simple: eat only wild food. Each participant then agreed to have their health markers and gut microbiome monitored.

The results suggested something remarkable,[34] but something that many of us foragers already suspected: that the wild diet, or The Wildbiome Project™, is one of the healthiest diets going. In fact, if this diet was rolled out across every country, we'd see a huge increase in the wellness of the population. One participant suggested, too, that it really helped her mental health. She was feeling rather depressed and flat beforehand and felt much more positive about the world afterwards.

What most of the participants had in common was that none of them was vegetarian, or at least, those that were chose to eat meat for the experiment. I'm sure that more trials will be replicated across the world and that, in the countries where it is possible, we will see people eating a vegetarian wild diet. Considering 50 per cent of my household is vegetarian, I can understand that this fact alone might be a sticking point for some who would otherwise try a wild diet.

But can you adopt this diet in a city? I wasn't so sure, so I called up my good friend Ru Kenyon, a participant of the wild diet study who lives on a boat in London. I asked him how he managed. He told me that he didn't hunt his own meat, he got a lot of venison from a hunter friend — exactly how I source all of my meat. Exactly how Dan Westall and his team organised themselves in their experiments with living in the Stone Age, too. It makes perfect sense to do so. Besides, there are laws regarding hunting animals in this country, and if you don't abide by them, you could face a prison sentence.[35] Running about with a bow and arrow in the wilds of Bulgaria for a TV show is one thing; running about central London firing arrows at pigeons is quite another. Aside from the practical reasons — like being arrested — it makes sense to have others doing the jobs you might not excel at, such as hunting.

Regarding foraging in London, Ru told me:

> I did forage mostly in London, which is pretty amazing, isn't it? The landscape has a cuisine and in that respect it is no different being in London than being anywhere else. The staples were venison, acorn flour, mushrooms — dried, pickled, and fresh. Then stored hazelnuts, walnuts, and dried fruit. Lots of wild greens. Also, the important other one was dandelion and burdock roots.

I quizzed him further about the roots, it being illegal to dig up roots in the UK unless you have the landowner's permission. Although dandelions and burdock plants grow in almost every public park in London and across gardens and allotments, too, he couldn't pick them. Instead, he travelled out to Essex and picked them on an organic farm:

> ... that was amazing, once you start to look at a field from a forager's eye view. It's just full of this valuable food, and the farm hates them. You do start to wonder about the calorific value that is just there ... People make these assumptions about foraging, that foraging couldn't sustain a group of people in the modern world. But no one has actually tested that. It's an assumption — it might be true, but we don't know ... I was in the woods yesterday picking some winter chanterelles ... I used to go there all the time just for mushrooms. But what I know now [after the experience of The Wildbiome Project™] is that that those woods are also full of pendulous sedge. A big seed crop, a massive seed crop in these woods. If you were someone who was living off

the land, you'd be going to those woods to pick those seeds more than you would be to pick the mushrooms. They are actually the most valuable food crop, calorically, that is in there.* It's like a field of pendulous sedge in there. You have to winnow the seeds; it's an art. You transfer them from one bowl to the next. It's mindful, it's nice.

This hits on a big snag when it comes to gathering and processing wild food: it takes time. According to a 2023 study, globally humans spend just six minutes a day processing food.[36] (Incidentally, we spend an average of one hour and six minutes of the day grooming.) Anyone who works with wild food will know that those jars of dried mushrooms, fridges full of fermented foods, sauces, and nut flour all take time to prepare. I've tried winnowing pendulous sedge and other seeds. I don't feel I have the patience, but Ru helped to frame it for me in a different way:

> You could spend all your time doing it [preparing wild food], as you can make more or you can make less. One thing that is very clear is that the amount of time you spend foraging is considerably less. The split is probably about 80:20. Also ... most of the things that people do all the time is pointless anyway. They may as well be processing wild food. When you are chatting, you

---

* Pendulous sedge (*Carex pendula*) is a native plant which is found in woodlands, especially damp woodlands. Occasionally, you might see it next to a sheltered path or making its home on the edge of a hedgerow. The long, sharp leaves grow up to about 1 metre (3 feet). It spreads rather rapidly and can cover the understory, making it abundant in the forests where it grows.

might as well be doing it while shelling acorns. The other thing is that it's going from being a chore to being something of a guilty pleasure. I actually enjoy doing it. It's satisfying and mindful. It's perhaps similar to what you want when you want to disconnect and scroll through your phone. You can do it in a procrastination way, for example. It's an escape. When you are putting off something that is more important, you think, I could just shell a load of acorns. That's the dream: to be somewhere that it isn't procrastination.

I asked if he was doing it now, and he told me that the bag of acorns is never far away. I admire Ru: he always seems to be pretty relaxed, a gentle soul who has pondered much about the human condition. He can offer a measured, thoughtful, and insightful comment on many aspects of life. I wonder if this is due to the fact that much of his downtime is spent processing acorns, rosehips, sedge, and whatever else is in season.

Ru lives on his own; he hasn't quite got round to trying to meet someone and seems perfectly content that way. My situation is very different: I've family around me, and much of my time feels like it is taken up with household chores, childcare, and earning a living. I wonder, though, if I am just telling myself that. Ru's comments came as a bit of a revelation. I thought about the time I have devoted to food preparation. About how sometimes we combine tasks: childcare with food preparation, for example.

Often, I find myself sitting around our kitchen table with my family. My daughter might be drawing or creating, Emma will be helping her or reading, my son painting his

Warhammer figures. I'll be stacking up the dehydrator, shelling acorns, deseeding rosehips or whatever. There is a gentle buzz about us, a quiet and easiness to the conversation. No pressure to speak. It feels natural and nurturing, and this is the time when our kids are mostly likely to share what is going on for them. To ask important questions about things that might be troubling them. Following afternoons like this, I feel fulfilled and nourished, and my sleep is always much improved. Ru and I talked about this, deciding that we should aim to have meet-ups where we prepare food in a group.

I'd debated joining in with the wild project. The idea of being part of the wilder group, of sharing food and recipes, seemed like it could be really rewarding. It turned out that I couldn't have been one of the participants of the wildbiome that year, as fate had something else in store for me. Emma and I found ourselves becoming the carers for a younger family member, Khloe,* who was growing increasingly ill. It was low level at first, and within the realms of normal childhood illnesses. But you can't leave a child on their own when they are ill, especially a young child. It's also hard to take them out and about with you when their energy levels are low — so the daily ritual of gathering was to be replaced by the daily ritual of care. She'd have a cough, a cold, burning sensations in her hands, fatigue — all things that could be explained by an online symptom checker or chatting with other parents ('Oh yeah, my kids had that too.').

That was, until we all planned a trip to Grannie's. 'I can't

---

* Khloe isn't her name, but I want to protect her identity and also to choose a name that means something. Khloe means young green shoot, something that is both delicate and strong.

breathe,' she said as I was reading her a bedtime story. Fuck. The ambulance was called, we rushed our way into hospital, and Emma spent the night with her while I looked after our offspring. A chest infection; a steroid injection and some antibiotics, and she was home. Full of energy. We felt like we'd dodged a bullet.

I had a window of time then in which to get out on my own and start enjoying the spring, to gather food to nourish and sustain us all. Seaweed is about the only vegetable Khloe will eat, and it felt good to be doing something positive for her health. I planned a trip to the coast to gather seaweed with friends. Foraging trips can be meditative and fulfilling when you go alone. Yet, when we come together to forage and prepare food, the mood is always buoyant. I frequently pick mushrooms with two friends, Rob and Alex, and it is simply fun. Our enthusiasm is infectious.

When we are on the hunt, I feel excitement from my belly to my feet. It can be rare to feel this sort of excitement in adult life; it's like being young again, a more wholesome version of following the string of voicemail messages to get to a rave: picking up on rumours, recalling hazy memories of past big hauls. I find my heart skipping a beat. For me, the prospect of mushrooms simply feels more exciting than other foods.

Come autumn, you start seeing flashes of mushrooms all over the place. 'You just have to get your eye in with these,' says Rob, slamming on the brakes and parking up like a drunk person. Out of the car he runs, returning with a cauliflower fungus. A huge mushroom that resembles a brain. We stay out picking until the light fades so much we can't tell the difference between a mushroom and a leaf. Rob drops me off to get a train home; the talk of the passengers is of fixed terms, pensions, and holiday allocations. It feels a world apart. I sit clutching a bag of hedgehog mushrooms, cauliflower fungus, amanitas, and various boletes. It's days like these when I feel tired and happy, with the richness of experiences making me feel wealthier than a billionaire — and I haven't even done a day's work.

I thought about that experience a lot while we were in the hospital, after things with Khloe got worse again. I thought about how nourished we'd all felt after it — how much my own kids get from being outdoors. How much I do. When I looked at Khloe, unable to do much more than sleep, with machines beeping all over the place and not a single natural thing in sight, I wondered if this experience could be offered on the NHS. Instead of car parks, or empty grassland, could we plant up the grounds of the vast hospitals across our country with fruit and nut trees? Could we let wild food plants grow, instead of thinking about spraying them with cancer-causing agents? Should we be planting birch, beech, oak, and pine trees, and encouraging the mycorrhizal fungi relationships not just around hospitals but across public land, perhaps even on failing farmland?

Imagine if the act of gathering food nourished us completely, not just nutritionally. Next time you walk down a supermarket aisle, imagine it's a forest. Instead of grabbing a bag of apples, you are plucking them from a tree. Instead of seeing kids melting down in a fake, sterile environment, they are happily playing. I'm getting carried away — this talk feels almost revolutionary, as it goes against our current order; I don't mean to be quite such an agitator.

But I do believe in the simple idea that maybe everything to do with food could nourish our spirits as well as our bodies, and perhaps even our communities, too.

NEW WILD YOUR LIFE

The first step in wilding your diet is to learn which foods around you are edible. There is a Further Reading section packed with foraging books at the back of this book, which will help you along the way. A physical guide will help, too — check the Further Reading section at the end for help with this.

It's easy, then, to incorporate a little foraging into your walks. Pluck the odd leaf or berry here and there, and snack as you walk.

Next, consider leaving the wild crops in your garden to grow rather than weeding them out. Look for areas that you might introduce a nut tree, or a fruit bush to supplement this. Consider reducing gravelled areas, allowing plants to grow between the cracks in your paving, or pulling up patios in order to give these crops more room to grow. I don't want to be the cause of any friction between you and those you live with, or your landlord, so I suggest chatting to them before making any major gardening decisions.

Live in a flat or don't have access to a garden? If you do have a balcony, consider that a root of nettles will grow happily in a container; a fruit bush, too. Alternatively, place a dandelion head on a pot of soil — any; they are not fussy — put it on a windowsill, and water it when it dries out. In a little over a month you'll have fresh dandelion leaves. Experiment with other wild plants, too.

When foraging seaweed, use scissors and don't pull directly from the rock, and be aware of the level of pollution where you are picking. Forager Mark Williams also offers the sage advice to tread between rather than on rocks when picking.

Foraging author Mo Wilde recommends using oarweed to replace lasagne strips, parboiling for 10–15 minutes first.

Seaweed Dip Recipe — by Rachel Lambert

Rachel is the author of *Seaweed Foraging in Cornwall and the Isles of Scilly*. She lives on the Cornish coast, where she forages and cooks seaweed daily.

This recipe uses an invasive seaweed called wireweed (*Sargassum muticum*) and is a doddle to make.

INGREDIENTS

- 150 g natural yoghurt or crème fraiche
- 3 heaped tsp dried and ground sargassum seaweed
- 1 tbsp lemon juice
- 1 tbsp virgin olive oil

Combine the ingredients and tweak according to your tastes. Let it sit for at least half an hour for the flavours to infuse. It keeps well for several days, too. Use as a dip with fresh bread or carrot sticks, or as a dressing over salad or cooked veggies.

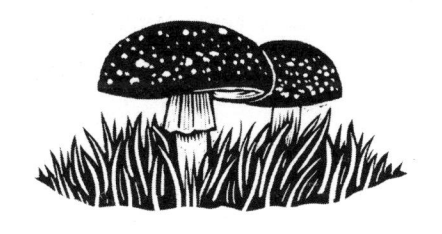

CHAPTER TWO

Consciousness

'The passionate desire which consciously or unconsciously leads a man to flee the monotony of everyday life, to allow his soul to lead a purely internal life even for a few short moments, has made him instinctively discover strange substances.'

LOUIS LEWIN, 1887

I want you to meditate for a moment. Close your eyes, focus on your breath and, while you are doing so, picture someone else meditating. When I do this, the first thing I think of is someone sitting cross-legged, preferably in the lotus position, atop a mountain with their palms face up — they may even be saying, 'Ohm.' This is certainly the image I had as a boy growing up in a new town in the middle of England in the 1980s. Back then, it felt as if meditation was something alien and mystical, not for the likes of me.

Besides, how could I clear my mind? Isn't a mind always on? Mine certainly was.

When I did start meditating, I felt like I had to be the best all the time, practically floating every time I tried, channelling the mountaintop Buddhist. For a while, in my twenties, I even hung out at a Buddhist centre, hoping that some of that Eastern mysticism would rub off — it didn't.

That was, until my good friend John Keen, who happens to be a Buddhist, passed me a short essay by His Holiness Dilgo Khyentse Rinpoche — his opening words dissolved the summit of perfect meditation that I'd created and replaced it with a far more negotiable plateau. I read: 'The everyday practice is simply to develop a complete acceptance and openness to all situations and emotions.'

I pondered this sitting — not cross-legged, I might add — on a train destined for London. I looked out of the window and took in everything I saw. I decided to tell my brain not just to be open but to *love* all I saw. The result was much like a dog must feel when it sticks its head of the window, smelling everything. I was overwhelmed with emotion; tears of joy fell down my cheeks. Luckily, the train was pretty empty. Since that moment, I've had more of an open mind when it comes to transcendental matters.

The more you practise something, the easier it becomes, and this is particularly true of meditation — it can start to increase grey matter in areas relating to memory, emotion regulation, and perspective, while increasing dopamine and serotonin.[1] The love of the areas that I forage and walk through has become a daily source of this sort of meditation: one of gratitude. It's been further enhanced with psychedelic experimentation.

'Frankly, the thought of doing anything that alters my perception of reality terrifies me.' Ray clutched his tin of stout a little tighter as he spoke and, with no sense of irony, punctuated his sentence with a sizeable swig. Ray had found ways to hide his awkward nature well in public and — just like many men our age, including myself — we'd both found beer helped to smooth out the edges of our social anxiety. Here we sat, in the local cemetery, above the war memorial to commemorate the dead. The sun was slowly setting and the memorial's shadow loomed in front of us, just as the wars still loom across men of our generation — people born of Baby Boomer parents. We are haunted by the shadows that our granddads' trauma cast over our own fathers. As the Kenyan proverb says, 'When the elephants fight, it's the grass that suffers.' Or to put it another way, when people fight, it's not just the fighters who are affected.

Both my grandfathers were brought up by men who had fought in World War I, both subsequently saw action in World War II, and both, I think, suffered from trauma. I've hazy, scattered memories of my maternal granddad; I was eight when he died at just 65 years old — younger than some of my close friends now. He was often out down the pub when we visited him and my grandma in Reading, or recovering in bed from a night of excess. If he came to visit us in Northampton, he'd be drunk when he and my grandma arrived on the coach. It was confusing for me as a young child: this slurring, beaming man felt a little dangerous to be around.

My dad's dad was a bit different. He was drunk a lot, too, but he also never quite grew up; we would say now his development was arrested. His favourite catchphrase was 'half my lies are true', so proud was he of being a pathological liar. It was very difficult to ascertain the truth from his fiction, yet through my nan we got something more closely resembling the truth. Some of the highlighted war facts were that he broke both legs, he always drank heavily, and his ship sank. He was either a hero or an unfortunate drunk. Most likely the latter — but, you know, he still went to war.

I want to believe that neither of my granddads were bad people. Certainly, neither did anything to *directly* harm me — in fact, other than passive smoking, it was just the opposite. Sure, when either of them had a penny to spend, it would always go on drink; they smoked, gambled, and had severe narcissistic tendencies — but could their behaviour have been a result of unresolved trauma?

If it was, they were not alone. World War II saw over 40 per cent of military personnel medically discharged from service due to psychiatric conditions.[2] Understanding of psychological problems such as post-traumatic stress disorder, or PTSD, was in its infancy back then. Much of it was still based on the half-baked theories of Freud, the coke-taking guy who thought everyone wanted to shag their mum. They suggested the soldiers were already emotionally flawed and that combat merely excited their anxiety levels.[3] Ironically, I can remember my paternal granddad talking negatively about his own *weaker* twin who suffered 'shell shock', something he was so deeply ashamed of that they never spoke.

Both my parents talk openly about their experiences growing up in these shadows. My mother: becoming homeless at 17 due to her dad's drinking; his cruel side, selling her toys to pay off his gambling debts, drowning her pet mouse in front of her. The physical and psychological violence my dad witnessed and was subjected to by his own dad. What they don't, and perhaps can't, speak of is how it affected them. Even my generation often struggles to talk openly of our emotions, a legacy left from the famous (and idiotic) British *stiff upper lip* culture of Victorian Britain,[4] which reached its zenith in wartime.

We might occasionally speak of how that in turn affected my emotional upbringing, but I don't feel we have to; instead, I'm content with thanking them for stopping the chaos of alcoholism and the cycle of violence and neglect. In fact, I'm quite proud of them, too. Given the trauma they both went through, especially my mum, they could have easily turned out to be pretty shitty parents themselves, but they really weren't.

I love them both for the life they gave me, for helping me become the man I am today. They have their issues, yes — but we all do. Although, I'm afraid to say (sorry, Mum), I have inherited some. The instability of my mum's upbringing meant that she suffers with anxiety; she tells me it was quite acute in my early years. I think this contributed to my own general anxiety disorder,[5] which was rather powerful in my early years and right up until my mid- to late twenties. I found it impossible to talk to groups other than close friends. Interestingly, I don't remember feeling anxious in the Scouts, especially when on a camp. I still have anxious times — they come and go — and I understand that overconfidence and anxiety are two extremes of my personality that I have to keep in check. This New Wild Order project has taught me that being outdoors, talking to friends, and disengaging from a screen all help. Disengaging from myself with psychedelics and meditation has also taught me that the extremes I experience happen when I allow thoughts to cluster. One anxious thought can lead to another and, before you know it, a whole cluster of brain cells have connected up around the same issue. I can choose to add to them or take a different route. I didn't know any of this at 14.

This was partly why I started drinking. Walking the streets near my home terrified me — although often with good reason, given where I grew up. It was the 1980s, so big worldly anxiety affected me, too. I often lay awake at night worrying about the threat of nuclear war, acid rain, the ozone layer, how overconsumption would destroy the planet, and if I'd ever get a girlfriend.

These might have been real issues that I had every right to worry about, but a small boy shouldn't have the weight of the world on his shoulders. It would often take me hours to get to sleep as I imagined the worst. So vivid was my imagination that even now the thought of nuclear winter creates a bitter taste in my mouth and a feeling of dread that I feel across my whole body.[6]

On reflection, I realise my family's — along with my own — issues resulted as part of the cycle of trauma. Just as second-generation Holocaust survivor Emily Wanderer Cohen writes in her book *From Generation to Generation*, 'the transference of trauma by the actual victims to their progeny is not limited to those who survived the Holocaust'.[7] Seventy million people served in World War II across the world, and many more experienced bombings and atrocities. That meant, for much of my generation, the trauma still hung in the air. Many of our parents had abusive parents; they lived in a world that dished out corporal punishment and everyday violence — a clip round the ear or a whacking with a slipper were all a fact of life, just as they had been for their parents and grandparents.

This violence became normalised, too, in my generation. The inequalities of a 1980s and early 1990s Midlands town meant we'd come through a time of violent race riots, miners' strikes, and football hooliganism. I'd often get beaten up on the way to school, or if I ventured into the wrong area at the wrong time. People brought knives, lump hammers, and other weapons into school; one older boy we hung out with had somehow managed to steal a police truncheon. These weapons were not just for show; they were frequently used. We also had interschool sectarianism, culminating in fights between Catholics and Protestants. I was never hurt — not badly, anyway. I narrowly escaped a stabbing and a few serious beatings, but it was nothing like a war; people didn't die and, apart from one stabbing at break time, everyone's testicles mostly stayed intact. Having said that, fairly frequently boys would be admitted to hospital, and the threat of violence hung over the town like a fart in a lift.

As I grew, something started to change. I believe that on some level there was a collective decision to break away from the trauma cycle. Those of us who were the children of Baby Boomers discovered the draw of recreational use of the drug 3,4-Methylenedioxymethamphetamine, better known as Ecstasy or MDMA. And Ecstasy started changing my generation for the better. We didn't just use it to dance; it also gave us something even more fundamental, something we were all craving — love and affection.

I can remember, at about 16, the exact words a close

friend used to describe a big acid house warehouse party: 'It's fucking brilliant — everyone is hugging each other.' We loved dance music, I fucking love dance music. I'd been drawn to it from the age of eight, when I first heard Herbie Hancock's 'Rockit'. Yet, we didn't talk about the music at all. We all got excited about hugging. We may not have fully admitted it to each other, but the biggest pull of raves for me and my friends was that you could hug a stranger. For people who rarely got hugged, it was a godsend. Drugs changed my town, they changed my life and, for a while, the effects were very positive. But alas, the party couldn't last forever. Around the mid-nineties onwards, I noticed a definite change. The love and empathy characterised by Ecstasy was replaced by the selfish culture that amphetamine and cocaine use bring. LSD became harder to find, Ecstasy was less potent, and speed was suddenly readily available. For the price of a pint, you could buy enough speed to last a night; what's more, it was a night that differed from a night of drinking, as you'd remember it all. You'd have energy, and it made you a better dancer — or that's what we thought, anyway. It was a high I fell in love with; the back of my neck still tingles with pleasure as I think about it. Needless to say, I indulged a little too often. Weekends bled into the week, and eventually there was more of the week when I was on speed than off it. I was even taking it to get up and go to work.

Mentally, this did me no favours. I'd have bouts of extreme delusional paranoia; nightmares plagued my waking hours. A reoccurring one had two of my friends appearing in my bed as demons who'd chew at flesh. I'd wake in pain and terror it was so real. A few months clean was enough to cure me, but for years it left a stubborn scar of paranoia. A scar that would rear its head when I was stressed. This was a problem I grew keen to address.

Two years after Ray and I sat at the war memorial, I found myself at our weekly online writers' meetings looking at Ray and the other members of our group. I hoped that one of them would ask how my week had been; everyone else seemed to be being asked. I was bursting to share. After my first week of microdosing, it felt like I had a secret that everyone should know, as though I'd stumbled across something that should be shared with all humankind. The group was keen to crack on, and the chance to talk about this new experience never arose. I was disappointed.

Maybe I was still a little high, too. Having read around the subject of microdosing, I'd been led to believe that it would be a simple affair. That I'd hardly notice any difference to my daily routine. I didn't find that at all to be the case.

It took me a while to come round to the idea that mushrooms were the medicine that I needed, that I craved. My bouts of paranoia were not terrible; I dealt with them by rationalising — a kind of CBT — and it worked. It was something else my brain did that bothered me.

Around ten years before, a relationship I'd had with a close work colleague had started to break down. Which is a polite way of saying that we'd have blazing rows — whenever we spoke either on the phone or in person — and I'd always find myself on the defence. This went on every day for months as I tried to untangle myself from them both financially and emotionally. I'm not going to assign blame — disputes are knotty, tricky things — but eventually, I realised that there could never be a resolution and they asked me never to speak to them again. I thought that seemed like a great idea and have stuck to it.

Yet, there were consequences to this decision. With no resolution to the arguments, my brain continued to argue. I'm not sure just how conscious I was of this, but every morning for ten years I'd stand by the kitchen sink and have a blazing row all in my head. It could leave me in a foul mood all morning.

I knew I had to do something about my dark moods. It feels ridiculous to me now, but I hadn't put together that my one-sided arguments had anything to do with them. A helpful friend of mine kept offering Mexican mushrooms — *Psilocybe mexicana* — but somehow this didn't sit right with me. Why try to eat local vegetables and then take drugs from far-off lands? If I was going to allow something to alter my brain, it had to be something that I'd picked, something that came from land that I was personally connected with, and something I knew had grown naturally. I had to make my own ritual.

My mushroom-foraging friend Martin offered to help. One morning, he set out to drive us to an unnamed destination somewhere outside Bristol — which could have sounded sinister if we weren't such good friends! As we drove, the claustrophobia of the city ebbed away, gardens grew in size, shops and houses became few and far between, and buses, taxis, and escooters totally disappeared, giving way to empty roads. Soon we were driving past the stone walls, open fields, and rolling hills of the Mendips. We ascended a hill, and the conifer and broadleaf tree cover thickened around us. It was a ten-minute drive, the distance of an afternoon's walk from the city, but it felt like we were in a remote wilderness.

Martin and I had bonded over our love of foraging

many years before. Since then, he'd become one of this area's most sought-after fungal foray leaders. Knowledge like that doesn't come without a touch of obsession, and he was already distracted by the surrounding mushrooms as his small Toyota wobbled disconcertingly along the stone track.

It was November, peak mushroom season. Up and down the country, foragers could be found scouring woodland and grassland, their eyes glazed and their thoughts solely on the hunt. Excitement bubbled, and it was infectious, with our fellow members of the Association of Foragers sharing their finds on social media. Each photo we'd seen posted felt like a drum was being hit for an ancient mushroom ceremony: faster and faster came the images of boletes, wax caps, parasols, and ink caps.

We darted out of the car like a couple of whippets and soon found a handful of ceps beneath the oaks. We took huge strides over boggy land until we reached the conifer woodland. With the thick carpet of needles dampening the sound of distant traffic, for once the constant hum that accompanies my life was deadened. The city was far from mind and body; it felt like a separate entity, a distant dream.

The air was the sort of damp that seems absent from the east of England, where I spent the first 25 years of my life. Here in the west we get persistent drizzle that eats away at your clothes and makes its way into your bones. But that is part of the charm of this world, a more comfortable world than the man-made, grey-edged world of the civilised. It felt like nature was bringing us in for a big-bosomed cuddle.

Our baskets grew heavier with the haul, and we stopped on a fallen tree to eat, an essential part of our outings. As always, each of us was secretly trying to impress the other with the food on offer. Martin produced an array of pickled wild foods and a health-giving mix of mushrooms in a tea, and I doled out my burdock-and-squash soup, flavoured with hogweed and served with freshly baked bread and some hand-churned, fermented butter. After filling our bellies, we moved on to our next competition: to make each other laugh. I'm happy to admit that Martin is always the victor.

Arising from the log for a moment to stretch my legs, I could see a tiny change of colour beneath the trees ahead. Amid the usual browns and greens of a forest, had I spotted some red? Could it be? Had I found what we had really come here for?

I made a beeline for a small plantation of conifers a few feet away. My suspicions were realised. Shielded by branches, but proudly standing beneath them, were a cluster of fly agarics, distinctive pillarbox-red toadstools covered with white warts. The trees they stood below were destined to be cut and used as Christmas trees. Trees that would slowly decay in someone's living room, adorned with baubles and ornaments. When we — humans — first brought these trees indoors, we dried the fly agaric mushroom on their branches. Our present-day ornaments that rest on these evergreens mimic that.[8] But I wasn't going to pick these mushrooms for ornamental purposes. No, I had plans for this mushroom, but I underestimated the plans that this mushroom might have for me.

Our ancestors used psychedelic plants, including plants that today we might consider deadly, to treat all manner of illnesses. Of these plants, the most widely used, venerated, and most documented are hallucinogenic mushrooms.

The earliest evidence of mushroom use takes us to the

arid desert of the Sahara — not the first place you'd think to look for moisture-loving mushrooms. However, if you had access to a flux capacitor–enabled DMC DeLorean or a Tardis, you could go back to the year 7,000 BCE and find the Sahara a very different place: considerably wetter,[9] and full of lush, verdant pastures grazed by giant herds of cattle. Ideal growing conditions, then, for mushrooms.

And grow they did. In a 9,000-year-old cave painting in the eastern Saharan country of Algeria, there are drawings which depict a visually striking, other-worldly image of what has come to be known as the *Bee man of Tassili n'Ajjer*. What makes the bee man particularly interesting is that he is holding a fistful of what appear to be mushrooms. In other drawings from the same cave, images of ancient dancers cover the walls. Is this evidence of a 9,000-year-old psychedelic-trance free party?

What might also be worth noting about this time was an event known as the Neolithic Y-chromosome bottleneck — that is to say, there was around one bloke for every 17 women. Some speculate that agriculture, which started to emerge 10,000 years ago, brought with it ownership. With ownership came war, with war came death and, generally speaking, it was the males who died.[10]

Another theory relates to a decline in the male birth rate. At this time, the world was warming and therefore changing dramatically. Ways of life handed down by generations could no longer be counted on: plants didn't grow in the same places, rains couldn't be relied on, and the game meat and birdlife may have disappeared as a result. Dental evidence suggests that during this time, 10,000 years ago, women were suffering from significant stress levels.[11]

Couple this with the many sources that suggest stress can reduce the male population at birth by a statistically significant amount,[12] as is seen in declining male birth rates after natural disasters or during the Covid-19 pandemic lockdowns,[13] and a picture starts to emerge.

One thing is certain: whatever was happening to the people of that time, it was unpleasant and lasted for generations. Something was needed either to stop the violence or to build their tolerance to change. Without the taboos and fear that have surrounded psychedelic use in our culture for years, perhaps mushrooms really did step in and make a difference.

If the bee man was an isolated case, then it might be considered a novelty, a quirk of societal evolution, but he wasn't. Countless other pieces of evidence suggest that drug prohibition is an abnormal state of affairs for humans. Mushrooms and other psychedelics have been used across the world throughout history.

In a cave lying between Valencia and Madrid in modern-day Spain, and thought to date to around 6,000 BCE, is another cave painting. This time we find an image of a bull with what looks like *Psliocybe hispanica* growing in the bottom corner of the image. These dung-loving fungi tend to grow in colder temperatures and have even been seen growing in snow. A suggestion, perhaps, that this mushroom could have even been used before the end of the last glacial period, also known as the Ice Age?

I can only imagine that those cold nights and long, long winters would have been made much more bearable with a fistful of hallucinogenic mushrooms to break the monotony.

There is also some speculation, from authors and

pioneering thinkers such as Terence McKenna, author of *Food of the Gods*,[14] that proto-humans were eating mutation-causing, psychoactive chemical compounds. Either by accident or with intent, the outcome was self-reflection and an enhancement of our information-processing activity. Perhaps it wasn't fire or meat that made us human, after all, but mushrooms.

Now that I have some experience with the fly agaric mushrooms, I can understand why a certain amount of ritual helps them to work. An open mind is essential to the experience. Of the dozen or so occasions I've taken fly agaric, each has been different. When it works well, I feel like I'm experiencing the personality of the mushroom. That she — and it does feel like a she — is taking me to a place devoid of language and showing me how to heal myself. I also think that the experience differs when you pick the mushroom yourself, and when you enter into it with respect for the natural world. I feel very protective over this mushroom and the land that it grows on. I feel like it makes me part of the land. Indeed, I have been almost reluctant to share my experience for fear that it could spark the destruction of this mushroom's habitat. That said, there is mounting evidence to suggest that harvesting mushrooms may actually increase yields.[15]

There is a long history of prohibition in the Western world. But now, psychedelics are gaining traction to become the new mental-health panacea. Various small-scale studies are emerging that suggest their benefits for those suffering from depression,[16] alcohol addiction,[17] and PTSD.[18] Yet, they are still dammed by many within our culture; indeed, I'm still not fully sure how my dad will react to this chapter. It's not just disappointing our fathers that we need to worry about, but the law. I can remember mushroom shops appearing across the country in the early 2000s, exploiting a legal loophole, only to be banned by a change in law in 2005.[19] Since 2016, anything psychoactive has been deemed illegal, including the fly agaric.

Yet, in recent years, the question of psychedelics has been turned on its head by medical professionals, researchers,[20] scientists,[21] doctors,[22] and psychiatrists alike,[23] all of them agreeing that there is high therapeutic value in magic mushrooms. Writers, too, are joining in the debate, such as Michael Pollan, who came to the party rather late in life: he was in his late fifties when he took psychedelics for the first time. He states that they are not for everyone, that those suffering from personality disorders or at risk of schizophrenia are advised not to go near psychedelics.[24] But his own guided trip saw him burst into a cloud of Post-it notes. With his ego dissolved, he felt more at ease with everything in the universe, and that consciousness is more evenly spread around the universe — leaves can gaze back at you.[25] The experience left him feeling that he didn't need to face the world with quite so many defences up as he had been.[26] He also stated that he would recommend psychedelics as important treatments for a whole host of mental illnesses.[27,28]

I was to learn later how to regulate the dose; instead, my first experiences of microdosing were rather unpredictable. One day, not much would happen — I might feel a little happier, a little dreamier, but nothing too out of the ordinary — the next, I'd be having a rather intense experience. I administered these doses by nibbling on a small amount of a cap dried in the oven. It wasn't exactly high-tech: I put the oven on the lowest setting, left the door open to allow the dehydrating liquid to escape, and just kept feeling the caps until they were dry.

Amanita muscaria contains two active chemicals, ibotenic acid and muscimol. The ibotenic acid is what causes ill effects, like vomiting, profuse sweating, and confusion. Drying converts about 30 per cent of the ibotenic acid, enough to tip the balance in favour of the muscimol, the chemical that causes euphoria, a dreamlike state, and hallucinogenic changes in perception.

The first time I took magic mushrooms, I took them at night. I figured if the trip was too hallucinogenic, I'd be able to sleep through it. I didn't sleep. I was visited by a feeling of femininity; I now describe it as a goddess, but in reality I'm just offering the closest thing I have to an experience that defies description. Whatever this thing was, it felt like this goddess had been sent to guide me, but the dreams she guided me into were not that helpful — they were too confusing and abstract.

Things weren't going well. I'd felt like I had been at last taking steps towards addressing the dark moods that had plagued me since childhood. Instead, it just felt like I was getting off my face, like I was chasing something of my youth. Taking drugs rather than medicine and doing it not to think. Then I remembered a trip I had taken during the day in my twenties. I can remember looking up at the clouds and falling in love with just how beautiful they looked. That it freed up my head for a summer. If I was going to take a natural substance, perhaps I needed to take it more naturally. I decided to switch and started taking mushrooms in the mornings. Each time, the same thing happened: I felt an urgency to be outdoors. When I stepped outside, I felt like I was stepping out into the Garden of Eden: greens were more vivid, the light was brighter, and the whole thing felt joyous; it was as if I was stepping out into a perfect spring morning. Places that were familiar became magical, tinged with a purple glow. I spent many pleasant days just like this; I'd often stop and just take in the beauty of the world — the familiar world in my neighbourhood. The feeling has lasted, too. After two years, I often just sit under a tree feeling totally at ease with the world.

When I did interact with people, I was a little odd, more so than usual. I'm pretty sure I was mostly harmless, however I did freak out the assistant at my local greengrocer's. She simply asked what I'd been up to. This stunned me, my mind filling with thoughts of the beautiful world I was inhabiting, but I couldn't work out how to articulate this — I thought perhaps she'd be able to sense it. She didn't; instead, she found herself alone in the shop with a silent middle-aged man smiling inanely at her for just long enough to be uncomfortable. She visibly recoiled on my next two visits, and I was flooded with guilt. I later explained that I'd been microdosing and suggested that I might have been acting a bit weird. In that very British way, I was assured that I hadn't been, and we returned to normal interactions.

The strongest and most profound experience I've had with magic mushrooms happened at home. My smartphone felt heavy in my hand, and then it started to feel like Salvador Dalí's melting clocks, the unsupported top and bottom parts bending downwards.* I felt that I couldn't

---

* At the time we were temporarily using a smartphone to stream music, but I could feel its addictive pull and have since got rid of it.

continue to hold on to it, that it was going to roll off my hand like a water-filled balloon. My psyche, the way I think, was now an abstract that I could observe. It was as if I was my own therapist and could think of and see my thought processes objectively. My brain knows that I respond well to humour and, like a good therapist, it gave me this feeling of my phone alive in my hand, which amused me greatly. I'd been poking away on it for longer than I needed to. Long enough for the mushroom I'd picked, dried, and just microdosed to kick in.

I'm a creature of habit, and there is a spot at the kitchen sink where I always ruminate. It's like my brain says: 'I know what we do at this spot. Here you go, have something negative to think about.'

When I ruminate, it can happen in two separate but similar ways. Either I have a one-sided make-believe argument with someone — anyone who, at that moment, I think has somehow *wronged me*. Or I go into full-on woe-is-me mode. This involves thinking about anything traumatic from my past. There are a few moments to pick from — not tons, but enough to fill a rather depressing after-dinner speech.

One day, though, guided by the mushroom, I did something different. Just as I intuitively knew that poking about on a phone wasn't doing me any good, I felt that this way of thinking had run its course. I stood by the sink, but instead of having an argument in my head, I was in a forest. I felt like the mushroom was sharing memories of the forest where it (she) had been growing. For the next few days, even without the mushroom in my system, I was back in that woodland every time I stood by the sink. I felt lighter, free of the heaviness of my own thoughts. I felt joy.

I'm pleased to say, that that joy has become a way of life, that I have felt lighter ever since.

I'd taken a small nibble of dried cap, a microdose of the fly agaric. According to life coach and fly agaric advocate Marianne Niklasson,[29] this is one of the best ways to take this mushroom in the modern world. She states that you can go about your day as normal when microdosing. I'm not totally sure; I always feel very light and giggly, and I was prone to stopping to admire the beauty of pretty much anything. I mean, I'm sure the parents on the school run think I'm an odd man as it is; for the sake of my kids, I really didn't want to fuel that any more.

I've since gone back to the mushroom on a few occasions. I've never taken what people call a 'shamanic dose', a dose large enough for me to have very vivid hallucinations and forget my own identity. I must point out that I seem to be either highly suggestible to the placebo effects of this mushroom or very sensitive to it. A couple of days ago, I took a standardised dose. It was less than half a teaspoon of a tea that had been made using a mix of different ground-down dried fly agaric caps, simmered for 15–30 minutes then strained. The caps are mixed so that mushrooms which are high in the active chemicals are balanced out by the ones that might be lower, making the dose more evenly distributed. Speaking to ten friends who took the same or a higher dose, I was the only one who reported hallucinations. Most felt pleasantly sedated, some even slept. I was awake for much of the night having some pleasant, but strong, visions.

This mushroom has profoundly changed me. My repetitive negative thoughts do sometimes try to arise again, but I feel like I'm getting further and further from that cave. I feel I'm letting joy into my life on a far more regular basis. Speaking to a close friend, who also happens to be a respected NHS therapist, I mentioned my experiences. Her response was astonishing: 'What you are talking about took me seven years of therapy.'

My subsequent experiences have not been quite so profound. They kind of top up the original feeling. However, I am somewhat alarmed, as I'm starting to hear anecdotal evidence coming from herbalists who have been suggesting this mushroom to their clients. They are indicating that there has been a noticeable increase in heart problems for those who have taken fly agaric. Perhaps there are other ways to reach the same state of mind. Time for some more experimentation.

My experience with the fly agaric got right into my brain, my daily functioning. If my brain were a river, it had been clogged by repetitive negative thoughts, as if a big tree had fallen into the waters, creating small whirlpools of negativity that swirled round and round. The fly agaric dislodged the tree, allowing the river to flow again. I felt like I'd been freed from my own self-generating negativity, and for quite some time I felt full of joy, but that was only part of the puzzle. I was gaining river management tools, but I had to be careful; the waters were still full of the detritus of my past and were starting to build up again. The mushrooms were fairly unpredictable; despite what some say, microdosing daily couldn't really be an option for me.

It was lovely spending my time gazing at the clouds,

but with the school run, household chores, and caring for Khloe as her condition deteriorated, I had to have my consciousness closer to earth and the people on it. Despite feeling more joy, it wasn't a joyous time, and these pressures were starting to build up.

I needed something. Magical thinking was setting in — I'd constantly throw a die; anything other than a six was bad luck. I knew it wasn't, but I felt compelled to fortune-tell like this. I also started to take longer dressing in the morning, as I had to decide which were my lucky boxers or lucky socks. These were thoughts I'd had since I was a teenager, but recently I'd started to realise that they were triggered by stressful events.[30]

Magical thinking is commonplace across cultures; it's the idea that we can influence events with just our thoughts. Instead of saying a prayer, blessing or an incantation in the morning, as many traditionally do, I turn to my lucky boxers. In fact, after admitting to myself that I need lucky boxers at stressful times, I've even started to bless them every day, like a prayer. I keep it secret from the kids, or at least I try to, but I suspect they've heard me. My daughter said to me the other day, 'Daddy, you like your pants, don't you?' I was too embarrassed to be honest and fumbled a 'Yes, they are useful things.'

One of the reasons this behaviour is so commonplace is that, as I've experienced, it is actually reassuring and helps to reduce anxiety levels.[31] It may even work on a physiological level: there is some evidence to suggest that blood sugar levels can be reduced by praying (though, just for the record, I couldn't find anything in the data about lucky boxers).[32] I reasoned that I was looking for reassurance and control in an otherwise unpredictable time. I was trying to write two books at once after years of focusing on bringing up the kids, putting writing on the back burner. I'd had a major health scare the previous year, which had seen me end up on a high dose of a medication that felt like it was poisoning me — which liver-function tests later confirmed.

On top of this, Khloe had got another cold. She might have been released from hospital, but that didn't mean she was better, and it didn't mean we'd stopped worrying about her. I was doing what I could do practically — shopping, doing the housework, checking finances — but I did not check in with my mind. I was around physically for the family, but I didn't feel I was around mentally — my son confirmed that recently, telling me he felt a distance from me at the time.

I go into myself when trouble strikes. Brain imaging suggests that this is a natural difference between men and women in times of stress.[33] I wanted to help and reassure my family, but instead I was distant, distracted, caught in a loop. When stressed, men tend to withdraw, and women are much more likely to do the opposite, seeking support from their friends.

I needed a way out of the loop. In the past, I might have continued in that negative, OCD state, but following my experience with the mushroom, I knew that I could detach myself from the anxious thoughts buzzing around my brain; I just had to find another way of reconnecting with my unconscious self. I didn't want to be distracted, sullen, and argumentative around my family. It wasn't really fair on them. I hoped, if nothing else, that a break would do me some good. I also knew from small fasts that I always felt great afterwards. Lighter.

Things were changing in my life: the kids were getting older and their needs were changing, and I was getting older, too, and becoming used to middle age. I feel like that's the time when you choose what sort of old person you'll be, when you address some of the habits or baggage that you picked up in early adulthood. Life is full of transitions, and it felt wise to be acknowledging that. Some kind of wilderness ritual felt like the right thing to do.

But what was there available for a white man of Scottish, Welsh and English heritage? A bit of digging about, and I found something about an utiseta.[34] An Icelandic tradition, the word translates roughly to 'sitting out', and it's a practice that was outlawed by Christians in the 13th century. It's similar to a vision quest. Both involve fasting and sitting out in the natural world in the hope of gaining insight or communicating with ancestors. However, I have problems with the modern vision quest — it feels like I'm stealing from another culture rather than honouring it,[35] and, as with the mushrooms, I didn't feel that medicine from another land was right. I wanted a practice from closer to home and found that in the utiseta.* Both the utiseta and the vision quest were practised when guidance was needed. Typically,

---

* The truth remains that I'm not Icelandic and so I am still stealing from another culture. In reality, these traditions have been outlawed for so long that we no longer have words in English to describe them; at best, we call them a psychotic break. Until a new word is coined, whichever language I use is going to be clumsy. I'm sure that I'll get some flack for practising this utiseta incorrectly; however, I fasted and sat by a crossroads, on what would be a waterfall in wetter weather. I did this at the start of the (pagan) year to gain wisdom, since the new year used to start in April. I chose to use the term utiseta as I'm a white European and can date my ancestors back to Scotland — maybe I did have some Icelandic in there somewhere? It felt right that I should call my practice something from white European culture.

it happened when people were transitioning from childhood to adulthood.[36] Aboriginal Australians also have a version, the walkabout, when young men from the ages of ten to 16 are required to live in the wilderness for up to six months.

When I was 17, I found myself in the Middle East. I had a flight booked to get home, but I didn't have any money for food, so I found myself accidentally fasting for a little over 24 hours. Back then I smoked, and so that helped, but I didn't remember it as a nurturing experience. It was painful, horrible; it felt lonely, too. Did I really want to repeat that?

My worries were escalating; I thought about getting hangry. I worried about being forced off someone's land in the middle of the night, about the cold — in fact, I worried about almost every little thing that could possibly go wrong.

My anxiety levels had reached a critical level. I needed to go, now, before I could change my mind.

I'd planned to drop the kids off at school and then go, by train, to Abergavenny in Wales, an hour away. There, I'd hike to the wildest spot my feet would take me. I didn't know where that was yet — according to Martin Shaw, author of *Wolf Milk*,[37] a book that reflects on two decades of running wilderness vigils, the place calls you. I hoped I wouldn't be too hungry to listen.

I decided to fast for 24 hours in total, from breakfast to breakfast, reasoning that if it didn't yield the results I wanted, I could always extend the experience at another point. I left my phone at home and bought a watch from a charity shop (they only had a women's watch, a dainty little blue number). I packed a tent, sleeping bag, and roll mat, and lots of warm clothes. It was April, but it had been cold.

As I walked to the train station, it felt strange being

disconnected from the world; I kept thinking of people I wanted to text or things I wanted to look up. After a while, though, these thoughts left me. My mind cleared.

What's interesting is that even now, over a year later, I don't feel any aspects of nomophobia.[38] I don't need to know where my phone is at all times; I often leave the house without it. Nomophobia (no mobile phone phobia) is an affliction which, according to one study, is thought to affect around 82 per cent of phone users, with 22 per cent suggesting that it is rather severe.[39] I am grateful that this trip severed my attachment to my phone, which had become another form of anxiety: I was always playing games, telling myself that if I got a certain score, things would be okay. Another form of magical thinking. Nomophobia is a real problem; it is suggested that it can negatively affect personality, reduce self-esteem, and increase anxiety and stress, while also reducing academic performance.[40]

I sometimes wonder how bad my mental health would be if I had kept my smartphone. I got rid of it when my son was just ten months old. I was in a cafe when I found myself staring down at it, looking at emails instead of my son's face. I looked over and saw another dad doing the same. The son, slightly older, was desperate for the dad's attention, but the dad barely acknowledged him. I couldn't help but wonder if I was acting the same and worried that I'd lose the real human bond I was developing with my son just to check my email.

The thing is, 92 per cent of all adults in the UK have a smartphone, a number that increases to 98 per cent of younger adults.[41] Globally, the balance has tipped, too, and now 4.3 billion people own a smartphone — that's over half the world's population.[42] And we are all glued to our phones, like I was.

As I sat on the train and looked out of the window, I felt at ease. I had a clear and simple goal: all I had to do was not eat, find somewhere to sleep, and put up a tent. I'd underestimated just how much this sense of purpose and clarity could help with my mental health; it is, after all, often put at the heart of mental health rehabilitation.[43] I pondered that the panic I'd felt about not eating had left. Yes, I was hungry, but I could observe the feeling rather than let it take over.

I'm often thinking about the next meal or what food I need to get in for the family — either foraged or bought. I can tell you exactly how much cheese we have in the fridge, how much bread we have, how many meals' worth of rice, when we will run out of milk, and how long the fruit bowl will remain full. These daily stresses were now removed. I felt like I was leaving another world behind. I still didn't know where I'd sleep, but that didn't worry me anymore. I pondered the idea of letting the world choose for me — what did that mean? Was I just replacing one form of magical thinking with another? Or would it be more like that call of the wild I had felt all those years ago in my back garden?

I decided that if I spoke to someone local and asked for advice, they were as 'natural' as anything in nature and therefore they could help me decide. Why not? I sparked up a conversation with the guy sitting next to me on the train heading out of Newport, Wales. After some chit-chat we found out we were both freelancers and bonded quite quickly. I told him what I was up to and he suggested that I should sleep on the Skirrid, describing it as a 'nearby mountain' which was 'pretty wild'. That'll do, I thought.

He asked me what had brought me to this point. I had to think of the sequence of events. We were both getting off at the next stop, so I said it was for something I was writing — this book. The truth was a lot more in-depth, much more complicated, and quite personal.

When I was 17, a few months after I arrived back from the Middle East, I had what doctors would describe as a psychotic break — not that I saw a doctor at the time. It ended up being the most transformative event I've experienced. I know for certain I wouldn't have become an author if I hadn't gone through it, but I also question whether I'd still be alive. The experience was a positive one, and it has carried me through some of the darkest moments of my adult life.

I was carrying a guilt that would have been a heavy burden for anyone of any age to carry. I believed that one of my friends had died because of my decision-making. In every quiet moment, I thought about him and how he'd still be alive if it were not for me.

We'd been out one night, drunk on cider and walking in the fields near his house in the early hours. Once we were out of eyeshot of the nearby estate, we happened upon a huge, muscular guy wearing a bandana. Who knows what he was up to or why he was there, but he whipped off his shirt and shouted into the wind, 'Who wants to party?' Innocently, naively, and dangerously, we both asked where the party was. This was the wrong response. He tensed his whole body, flexing biceps the size of barrels, and then repeated the question. This time with a growl.

We ran.

'Split up,' shouted Doug, knowing Barrel-arms couldn't catch us both. He ran after Doug, leaving me to escape.

I saw the fist flying through the air, then heard the thud against Doug's head, closely followed by his cry ringing out across the fields. He fell to the ground. The guy took Doug's watch and scarpered. I was a safe distance away and managed to raise the alarm to get the police out.

Later that winter, Doug died of a brain haemorrhage, and I felt responsible. I reasoned that I should have tried to stop the guy, that we should never have walked out somewhere so obviously dangerous. Clouded by grief, others condemned my actions and blamed me for his death. If what happened next was a psychotic break, then this level of shame and guilt would have no doubt contributed towards it.[44]

Doug had lived for a summer in a caravan in Cornwall, and shortly after his death a friend and I stayed there for a week. Over that week, we both felt his presence, right there in the caravan. Perhaps this was nothing more than a hallucinatory state — it's not uncommon for people suffering bereavement to have hallucinatory experiences, after all. In a 1971 study published in the *BMJ* entitled 'The Hallucinations of Widowhood',[45] almost half of all the people interviewed experienced what the medical profession calls hallucinations, manifesting in the form of visits from their dead spouse or loved one. Hallucination or not, I wanted this feeling. I missed my friend and feeling him nearby helped.

So I returned to the caravan with the same friend and one other, but ended up arguing with the second friend about a girl we both liked. I found it hard to stick up for myself back then. Instead, every time I got pissed off, I'd go on a walk.

Back then, I had the sense of direction of a moth in a room full of bright lights, and so a short walk away from our campsite meant being lost for hours on end. I walked far and wide, mostly at night and mostly around fields of green, immature wheat, and up and down the thin country lanes with high hedgerows that characterise the south-western tip of England. I barely ate, not because I wanted to fast — I mean, I didn't really have much of a concept of that — but mostly because I was young and rather inept. I had little idea what effect this would have on me; it was in no way intentional. As I walked, I was lonely and scared at times. I phoned the police at one point. They were initially willing to come out and help me find my way back, but they dismissed me as a crank when I asked them to bring cigarettes.

On the third night of walking, I found myself in the middle of a thunderstorm. All the time I still felt I was seeking something, that I was out with a head full of questions. The dark night was flashing white, and the rumble of thunder bounced off the cliffs, echoing and foreboding. I must have been in the eye of the storm, as I don't recall getting wet at all — maybe I was already too far gone. I felt electrically charged, elated. The scene was set for some kind of psychological experience. I stripped to the waist and put my T-shirt over my head like a headscarf. Hallucinations had been kicking in; earlier that day, I'd seen myself in the campsite mirror, and an image of Judas Iscariot looked back at me. Now, for a moment, I felt that I was him.

It was then that the police decided to show up. My eyes were wide, crazed, reflecting the enormity of feeling that

I was going through. They asked if I was okay, and added, 'Because you do look a bit odd,' and, 'You can see why we stopped you.' I still don't know why they didn't section me there and then. I somehow managed to agree that I looked odd and send them on their way, kicking myself for not asking for a cigarette.

The dark clouds of the storm hampered the morning twilight, and it was then that my hallucinations intensified. The fields around me went black, like a never-ending stretch of tar sands. I felt grief like never before. Tears rolled down my face; I was distraught. I cried out. I felt I was witnessing the end of all life on our planet.

Then, just as the sun rose across the horizon, I saw a single yellow flower. I wiped my eyes. Then I noticed another, and another, and another. Soon the whole landscape was awash with yellow. My tears were now tears of joy — joy like when your children are first born.

I continued to walk. The sun was now bright in the sky; morning had reached me again. I felt a presence next to me — not Doug this time but a stranger, a loving presence, I think a man. I smiled at him and felt the return smile. I felt like whoever was next to me would be with me always. But then I felt the same on my other side; another person was there too, and they were smiling, supporting me; and someone was next to them, smiling too. I spun around, and people were everywhere, all supportive, all joyous. I felt like I was part of them and they would all help me. I returned to the caravan changed.

The events over those three days were something of a rite of passage, a transition from boyhood to manhood. My brain somehow conspired to give me exactly what I needed at the time it was needed. Was this a psychotic break, or was it a moment of spiritual awakening?[46]

I felt like life's purpose was to spread happiness. Soon after, I started writing — mostly terrible poems that I thought were deeply profound, but also comic books, the plots to stories, and the outlines to films. Moreover, the positivity of seeing the end of the world and the subsequent regrowth of a new world gave me something else — hope. Hope that has helped me through many tough moments, including the deep depression I went into afterwards as I tried to make sense of it all.

Other major events came to test me. In my early twenties, I realised I had a problem with amphetamines and gave them up cold turkey. My brain had been battered by the drug, causing temporary damage to my dopamine levels.[47] I was unable to feel excited, and became very low for over a year, suicidal. I barely left the house during that year. I was broken and empty, and suicide felt like the only way out; I thought about it on a daily basis. Sometimes I'd hold a knife to my arms, other times I'd hold a bottle of pills in my hand. Each time these intrusive thoughts threatened to take over, I'd remember the image of that field of yellow flowers and the joy of being surrounded and supported by something other than myself. It was an image that stayed with me and helped me through.

It's since got me through periods of loneliness in a new city, housing insecurity, the worst of the lockdowns during the pandemic, and climate crisis worries. And, after those days in Cornwall, my childhood worries about nuclear war never returned.

In every way, it was the most important few days of

my life, and it happened just as I was becoming an adult; it gave me a purpose, and then it kept me alive to achieve it. But as useful as it was, there isn't a place for an experience such as this in our current culture, and it often feels like I have to keep the whole thing to myself. I've had attitudes towards me totally change when I tell people about it. I'm treated with distrust, fear. I sometimes get asked, 'How's your mental health now?' I can understand why; I've also rationalised the experience as a psychotic episode — it's easier than suggesting that something spiritual happened. Psychotic symptoms in themselves are not uncommon, especially for young people: they occur in 17 per cent of all nine-to-12-year-olds and 7.5 per cent of adolescents aged 13 to 18.[48] That's about two or three children in every classroom. All of us will know someone who went through a psychotic break of some sort, if we didn't go through one ourselves.

Then, in preparation for this book, I started reading about the cross-cultural and sometimes religious practice of fasting in nature. The ancient Norse would practise utiseta sitting on sacred ground and communing with their ancestors.[49] Religious texts are littered with the idea — it's almost as if they are trying to tell us something. The Old Testament has Moses fasting before he went up the mountain,[50] and in the Christian Bible Jesus is tempted by the devil.[51] In the holy book of the Quran, 'fasting is prescribed for you as it was prescribed for those before you, that you may develop God-consciousness'.[52] The Buddha is thought to have gone out to the forest and fasted,[53] encountering supernatural beings,[54] just as I was hoping to. Throughout history, others have experienced a similar moment,[55] some sort of transformation, a death of the old self and rebirth of the new self, just when they needed it.

Now, in middle age and with new responsibilities weighing heavily on my shoulders, I felt like I was again in need of some direction, or at least good mental health for the next stage of my life. I needed to follow the call of the wild once more.

I got off the train and the guy pointed me in the right direction for the Skirrid. Looking at my map, it was more of a hill than a mountain, and it didn't seem that far from civilisation — I mean, there was a cafe and a car park at the bottom of it. Was this really the *right* kind of wilderness? I repeated what I'd been telling myself: I could always just treat this as a test run should I not find what I needed. I'm not sure I even really knew what I needed.

As I walked, I started to get hungry, really hungry; for the first time ever, I was annoyed that I knew so much about which wild plants are edible. I sat under a lime tree — *Tilia cordata*, a tree with edible leaves. Next to it grew Jack-by-the-hedge — *Alliaria petiolata* (edible) — and blackberry shoots — *Rubus* — still green and very edible, a great little snack. It was torture.

I poured myself a tea and breathed through the hunger. It didn't work. I reflected that I was the worst person to undertake a fast; I loved my food far too much. I was always snacking. Even when out walking, I'd be snacking on plants. At this time of year, it felt like everything around me was edible: hawthorn leaves,[56] ground elder,[57] wild carrot,[58] lesser celandine,[59] which has edible raw leaves before flowering (they weren't), young dock leaves, [60] edible when young (they were), dandelion,[61] field mustard,[62] daisies,[63] and hairy bitter cress.[64] Why on earth had I decided to fast during one of the tastiest times of year for wild food?

I crossed a golf course and saw a sheep bleating at me on the other side of the stile. I looked at her lambs and in my mind's eye I saw lamb chops sizzling under the grill. They were no longer animals but food.

'The place will call.'

I was starting to think that was total bullshit, but then I felt a pull, a call from a nearby brook. I ignored it at first, returning to the map to follow the way I thought was right — the rational way that I'd planned with a rational mind. I looked at the map again and realised this short diversion would save me from lugging my heavy backpack all the way up a steep slope; the pull made sense even in a rational way. Was this the place calling me?

I had felt the same sense of guidance when I had taken the mushrooms. It reminded me of the pull of a repeated rhythm on a drum. I'd also experienced it when coming off high-strength steroids in the Vallée des Merveilles in Mercantour National Park in southern France. My strange experiences were starting to weave themselves together, and they were taking me down some very real paths along with some very unexpected and surreal paths within my mind.

Was this the same pull? Was it a kind of madness? I'd barely started to walk up the hill when she (once again, it had become a she) beckoned me down a small path. Then, right in front of me, there was a shelter — a fucking shelter made around a fallen tree. There was no way I'd have found this myself. What was going on?

The shelter was in a dip on the hill caused by an old

river; it sat on a small mound, and despite being less than 10 metres (15 feet) from the crossroads caused by two main paths, it was hidden in every direction — exactly the right ground for an utiseta. I put up my tent inside it, and it fitted perfectly.

My notes from then on were mostly about food. I did conduct some sort of ritual; I'd read that it would help. It felt odd, and I was half arsed about it. 'I bless the ground,' I said in a mocking voice while walking a 'sacred circle'[65] around the tent, waving a feather about. Oddly, this did make me feel safer. I guess it was the right kind of magical thinking! My shaman friend, Sam Hobson, later told me that ritual speaks to the inner brain.

As the sun set, I decided to walk further along the Beacons Way — the nearby footpath. I wanted to see the moon or the sunset; I mean, why shouldn't I make the most of this? I wasn't about to just sit inside a circle for hours.

I felt like a naughty child as I walked up and around the hill, a feeling that soon ebbed away as I found a great spot, flat and with plenty of tree cover, where I could see out across the valley. As I approached the area, though, I heard a deathly noise. It was the noise of a fox warning me off;[66] at this time of year, she would be protecting her young.[67] When I returned to my camp, I felt that I was returning to myself. To my spirit. That part of me would always be part of that hill.

I went to bed early that night, an hour after sunset. I wrapped myself in three layers of clothing and a sleeping bag, and I slept.

In the middle of the night, I got out of the tent and looked up at the stars; they twinkled as if to say, 'Hello, welcome back.' I now felt part of them. Then I looked at the trees. They looked like giant strands of kelp with shrubs of carrageen and other seaweeds surrounding them. I was at the bottom of the sea, and it felt fun. The whole forest seemed alive and full of fun. I was part of it now.

I stayed looking up from the sea floor at this sight for a while, until the cold and bitter wind-chill drove me back into my tent. When I awoke the next morning at 5.15 am, I felt elated. I'd almost done it; it wasn't long until I would have gone 24 hours without food. I realised I hadn't thought about cutlery and didn't have anything to eat my breakfast with, so, for the next couple of hours, I set about carving a spoon from a tree branch. When finally I started to eat my muesli, my jaw ached; I guess as I hadn't used it. With each mouthful, I started to return to the self I was used to; I felt that I'd been elsewhere for a while.

After packing up, I walked down the hill and pondered the meaning of my utiseta. Sitting on the train on the way home, I felt content, at peace with myself in ways that I really hadn't the day before. I looked around, and everyone I could see had earpods in and was tapping away at their phone. I wondered if any of them were suffering like I had been 24 hours earlier. I wondered if any of them needed their own hill to rest on.

I walked back from the station and arrived home; I felt immediately present with my family. I wasn't distracted and could be around for them emotionally. Over the next few days, Khloe reached another crisis point: her health took a nosedive, her energy levels plummeted, and her legs got weaker, becoming too weak to walk. Emma called me from the doctor's. It was serious.

It's not a call that anyone wants to take. It felt like I was underwater; my brain couldn't quite process the magnitude of it. The world around me quietened, and only that moment existed. It was like the shock of grief.

We took it in turns to stay at the hospital with Khloe. CAT scans, lumbar punctures, and a host of tests were done. The nurses have to look out for signs of neglect, and so we felt under observation.

The room we sat in was a few storeys up, the view was out onto a brick wall, and the food was as good as mass-produced food on a tight budget can be — that was, unless you could afford the expensive Marks & Spencer food court in the basement (we couldn't). The whole experience was stressful and the polar opposite of what we actually needed. This is where I want to say how great the nurses and doctors were, but apart from the occasional real human moment, they all seemed under pressure in a system that has been underfunded and broken for years. It wouldn't be fair to moan, as I think they were all doing their best, and it was no different than when I worked for the NHS.

When we left hospital ten days later, we had no real clear diagnosis, just an idea of what might be going based on what it wasn't.

Had I not been on my utiseta, I think I'd have spiralled with anxiety and retreated further into myself. I'm not sure how well I'd have coped inside the hospital, especially while feeling like I was under observation. Instead, I stood back and focused my attention on where it needed to be — I could help. I could be human to the nurses, the doctors. Work out what was best for the child we were looking after. We eventually got the diagnosis of chronic fatigue. This was going to be a long journey with no real endpoint, and thankfully I was in a good place to deal with it.

Fasting and being out in the wilderness had given me strength and guidance just when I needed it. I'll repeat it one day, if I need to. Practising my own utiseta showed me why it appears in so many different religions and cultures. But the fact remains that any form of spirituality is diminished in the Western mindset; often, it's dismissed as psychosis,[68] a diagnosis that I know doesn't help anxiety levels or self-esteem. I know that when I've shared my experiences with some of my friends, although some were quite accepting and intrigued, others ridiculed me, and some even worried for my sanity. These are natural reactions to something that challenges our entrenched view of the world.

I was starting to enjoy my journey back to the wild; it was bringing me closer to my family and myself. It was helping undo some entrenched patterns of behaviour. I'd also lost a few pounds. Crazy had never felt so healthy.

NEW WILD YOUR CONSCIOUSNESS

There's plenty of literature out there on meditation — the only thing I'd like to add is to say that it's not a race. You'll get better with practice; just start with appreciating all that you see.

If you are planning to microdose, I'd suggest talking to someone else who has tried it first. Start on a very low dose and work up. If you have a therapist, talk to them before and after. Always know the source of your mushrooms. Avoid taking them with other medicinal and street drugs; if you are pregnant or suffer from schizophrenia, you should also steer clear.

Work up to the amount of fasting you are comfortable with on an utiseta; try a fasting window of 16:8 hours and increase this to 20:4 hours for a couple of days. Avoid driving and heavy lifting during those days. It's also wise to bring along a friend for your utiseta. Still conduct the ritual alone, but designate an area where you can leave a sign for your compadre every hour, such as a pile of rocks or a niche etched into a fallen tree. Listen to your intuition throughout and use that as a guide.

You know yourself well enough, but I'd seriously consider avoiding fasting if you have an eating disorder.

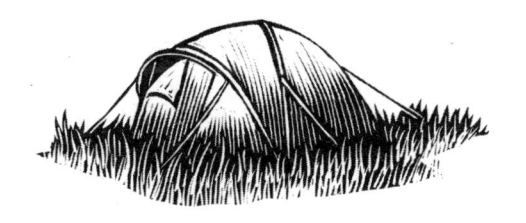

CHAPTER THREE

Shelter

'I have been bent and broken, but — I hope — into a better shape.'
CHARLES DICKENS, 1861

According to author of *The Great Indoors*, Emily Anthes,[1] North Americans and Europeans spend about 90 per cent of their time indoors. With online grocery shopping, and courier services collecting our parcels, even short trips outside can become a thing of the past. As a writer, there can be times where I spend far too long in front of a screen at home. I'm not alone, and remote working has become the norm, with around 40 per cent of us working from home at least once a week.[2] According to the World Health Organization, this not only affects our mental health but our physical health,[3] too, with an increase in obesity levels and all its associated problems.

My time practising the utesita has made me want to

address that. I've also started to notice that my knees click when I stand, my back hurts more often than it should and, worst of all, I've started saying 'oof' when I get up from the sofa. Not only have I started to feel old, but I feel like a fraud, like I've started to spend more time writing about an outdoor lifestyle than actually living it. I'm also certain that my shelter and how I live in it is making me ill. Time for some changes. The first step: to get a hammock.

Which is why this morning, about half an hour ago, I sat out in my newly acquired hammock, sipped some tea, and looked up at the sky and the leaves on the apple tree. Since putting it up, I've really started to cherish my 'hammock time', a time for me to sit and daydream whenever I need to. It's a new practice that I've adopted, and it's helping to keep me happy. You see, if I'm not careful, a typical weekday can start at 7.00 am with the making of breakfasts and packed lunches, and end at midnight, when the kids finally go to sleep — part of the irony of chronic fatigue is that you can suffer from insomnia.[4] If I don't grab these moments, I can get lost in a whirlwind of endless tasks and not have much rest in a day. Then I get grumpy.

But today, instead of moving into a trash can and becoming Oscar,* I gently rock in my hammock and ponder the coming harvest; it's August, and the summer is calming down. I look up at our apple tree — it's been a barren year, and only one apple sits on its branches. My mind gently wanders, and I think of all the apple trees that are and have ever been. I think of the rhythm of the apple season and imagine a long line of happy pickers reaching back through

---

[*] The grumpy guy who lives in a trash can on *Sesame Street*.

time; these gentle thoughts leave me feeling nourished. I sit in this part-dream world for a moment, seeing the apple workers fill my garden as they sip cider and laugh. That is, until the siren from an ambulance throws me back, with a jolt, into the city soundscape, into the reality that is modern urban life.

We are sandwiched between the main trunk road that leads in one direction to Somerset and in the other to Bath, and unfortunately sirens are a near-constant noise menace. The siren is closely followed by two pigeons who shoot across the sky a couple of metres above my head, one heading east to west, the other west to east. The words from countless ads ring in my ears: 'We've all got busy lives'. I ponder the lives of millions of commuters rushing about in cities across the world. Are these pigeons really that different? I then wonder what a corporate pigeon might look like, and smile to myself at the thought of its tiny tie, polished shoes, and briefcase tucked under its wing.

It's the school holidays, and it's been wet, so most of the time I am indoors. I often wonder if the thing that really helped me on my utiseta was the time spent outdoors. I crave time to have thoughts about corporate pigeons and mini briefcases, and this morning I needed that time more than ever. I've been feeling a little down for a while and I didn't sleep well last night. Between family troubles and work troubles, there has been a lot going on. Before the holidays, I was keeping things in check; I felt happier after my utiseta and was able to deal with these normal life pressures. I indulged myself with a walk across the local wild cemetery as often as I could and attended the Human Nature Project once a week, a forest bathing session run in

Leigh Woods, the two-square-kilometre forested area over in the north of the city. It was helping me, and it seemed to be helping many others.

I'm ashamed to admit I was a little sceptical when I was introduced to the concept. A forest bathing practitioner told me that trees have different personalities. I nodded politely and pondered what other rubbish she might spout, as we walked around stopping at every cluster of trees to look up. At first, she described the differences between the clusters, urging me to listen to the sounds, to take my shoes and socks off and feel how years of leaf fall creates mulch that differs from place to place. She told me to take a deep breath and take in the smells. This woodland was managed, and so there were clear variations in the planting: poplar, beach, pine, oak, and even a patch of yew. After a while, I too started to notice the different personalities of each area, as if we were tasting whisky, cheese or an aged fine wine. Perhaps she was on to something, I realised.

Without any scientific training, she had intuitively taught herself how each tree, and the soil it grows from, can positively affect us. And she was right. Just an hour in the woods can help to stimulate a host of neurochemical responses, such as increasing serotonin,[5] the happiness chemical that can also help you sleep. It can lower blood pressure,[6] and increase the amount of beneficial, cancer-busting natural killer (NK) cells we produce.[7]

My keenness to try this again, years later, helped me to find Sam Hobson and Ava Maginnis. In their sessions, they had us look at the way the light shone down through the leaves on the ground, searching for movement and listening to the sounds of the forest, each focusing a different part of our awareness. Our guards were down and so, at the end of the session when we were all seated in a circle, we shared more than we might have in an unnatural setting — such as a conference room, church hall or office. By the time we'd reflected our thoughts back as a group, it felt like there were no barriers between us; we were all speaking with a rare honesty. Many reflected on their lives, from recent bereavements, to disillusionment at work, divorce, and many other problems. We found some togetherness there in the woods; it was a real tonic made all the stronger for being in a group. In many ways, I felt like I was reliving some of the camaraderie that I experienced in the Scouts. With the added benefit that perhaps the forest was helping to facilitate these bonds.

Then came the school holidays, and my focus had to change from myself to my family. Trips out were difficult with Khloe still in a wheelchair. I was also falling behind on many deadlines. When I'd been feeling a little low for a week or two, I tested myself on the — seemingly eponymous — Hamilton Depression Rating Scale. The test suggested I was suffering from moderate depression,[8] not for the first time.

It is no secret that I get low moods; I have done since childhood. They intensified in my late teens and early thirties, sometimes confining me to my house, where I'd shun anyone close to me, anyone trying to help, feeling that I was unworthy of their time.

These days, I see my moods as something different, as a time to reflect. Low moods can be a sign that I need to eat, get a decent night's sleep or go for a walk. Longer and darker moods are the makings of a depressive episode, where something more major is going on. I believe that depression can be a strong indicator that something is very wrong in our environment. We live in a world that is overfed but malnourished, sunlight deficient, overly competitive, sedentary,[9] and sleep deprived, after all. It's a wonder we aren't more depressed!

When I reflect on my more major depressive episodes across much of my life, I notice a pattern emerging. During these times, some or all of the elements in the magic triangle of work/purpose, home, and society/friendships were missing or vulnerable. During each of the episodes, my mood was further confounded as I spent more time indoors, fearing the world outside.

Access to greenery, I've learned, is crucial for my wellbeing. It was one of the reasons we moved to this house, which has access to a green space. But I have to ensure I actually go there, and so I have built in a set route and routine. At least once every two days, I walk the 500 steps from where I now sit until I'm out among the trees on the edge of our local park. I take this in, along with the view of the Cotswold hills. I then walk another 500 steps, and I'm sitting on a bench in the middle of the wooded Victorian cemetery, Arnos Vale.

Sometimes I sit and watch the squirrels making their homes — known as drays — or I might grab a drink from the cemetery cafe and sit and look at the greenery. I'm not the only one who does things like this, and the need to be outdoors has been recognised since the 19th century,[10] when parks started to emerge in Britain.[11] Indeed, it wasn't just here, but over in North America, too, and in 1857 the landscape designer Frederick Law Olmsted started work on Central Park. Drawing on his extensive experience and observations, his own research, and his links with the asylum reform movement, he noted that city dwellers suffer from a whole bunch of maladies, including nervous tension, over-anxiety, hateful disposition, impatience, irritability, and other symptoms.[12] That they (we) need to 'withdraw the mind to an infinite distance'.[13]

Author and Professor of Environment and Society at the University of Essex, Jules Pretty, agrees, stating that we've been close to nature as hunter-gatherers for 350,000 generations.[14] No wonder time without nature makes us feel gloomy.

Yet, my favourite take on our need for green spaces goes back much further in time and comes from storyteller and mythologist Martin Shaw.[15] Being a storyteller I'm not sure how much artistic licence he's employed, as smoke holes would often be shut during inclement weather and the term *Siberians* covers a variety of people and cultures – still, the imagery holds up and it's a great image. He tells us that if the Siberians wanted to hurt someone, they would sneak inside their tent and close their smoke hole. This would cut them off from the outside world — the natural world of mountains, rivers, lakes, and forests — leaving the tent's inhabitant alone with just their neurosis for company.

I'd had my own neurosis for company for too long, and my self-diagnosis of moderate depression simply confirmed what I already knew. I wasn't about to let it progress to severe depression and the anxiety that often comes hand in hand with this. So, where to go to withdraw the mind to an infinite distance?

It was late August, when Emma always takes the kids up to Scotland to spend time with her family in her sister's small flat. I usually stay at home, giving me a week to catch up on work, do DIY or restore myself. This year, I really needed to restore myself — a glance at my shoddily put-up bookshelves, barely holding the weight of the books on them, reminded me that both the DIY and my work would benefit if I took time off.

The stage was set for an extended forest bathing session. These days, Olmsted's work has been furthered by Dr Qing Li.[16] Li is an author and proponent of *Shinrin-Yoku: The Art and Science of Forest Bathing: how trees can help you find health and happiness*. Li's prescription to any overly anxious or fractious city dweller is three full days in a forest. This would also help me to sleep better, become less aggressive and grumpy, and improve my immune system by increasing the number of NK cells produced in my body.

The law had recently changed in England, so I couldn't camp wild without fear of being arrested. I thought about going to Sweden or Scotland, two places where friends have access to woodlands. However, a lack of time and money dictated that I should camp out in my friend John Atkinson's small woodland, just on the edge of Bristol, within a half-day's walking distance, or about six miles (9.6 kilometres), from my home. Half the population of England also lives within six miles of woodland, so this seemed appropriate.

John's site is a two-acre plot that backs onto the larger expanse of Leigh Woods. This meant I had somewhere to sleep and a wider area of woodland to roam in during the day. I decided to stay for four nights, just to ensure I got a full three days' camping experience. I'd leave my phone at home and only pack two books and a notebook for my entertainment. I figured I'd try to have as much hammock time as possible. I wanted to grasp some of what I'd felt during the utiseta; I was keen to experience some calm without the need for starvation. I felt like I'd made a great deal of progress with my own mental wellbeing, that I didn't need any big revelations that came with utesita or mushrooms. I mean, it would be good to have an activity that calmed me, that I could also share with the kids and Emma.

The day I arrived, I was a little giddy with excitement, and I took off all my clothes and ran around naked for a while. I'm still not sure what came over me — I think it must have been the freedom of being on my own. One of the dads on the school run once asked me if I got naked when I wild-camped. I wasn't sure if a) he was living vicariously through me, or b) he was rather fond of the idea of me naked in the woods. However, I thought perhaps c) was the most likely.

c) He was taking the piss.

I might have been naked, but there was work to be done. I put up my two hammocks — this was rather a pertinent idea as, due to the mild summer and abundance of deer, the woods were riddled with ticks. I then placed a tarpaulin over one of the hammocks for my shelter and put up a tent to house my bag.

My mood was already lifting. There are studies to back up the (rather obvious) conclusion that a break from the daily grind will help raise one's mood.[17] There is seemingly little need for studies such as this, yet they do help doctors to consider prescribing a holiday as a real alternative to anti-depressants.[18] The break from my parental and caring responsibilities was a huge help, and I vowed to make sure Emma got a break soon, too.

During that first day, I thought about how different

this place was from my normal everyday life. All I had to do was be there, stay hydrated and fed, and keep warm. On that note, I put my clothes back on, lit a fire, boiled water, and started to cook my dinner. I didn't need to nip off and do five other things — instead, I could check on the fire from the comfort of my hammock, treating it as if it were a sleeping baby.

As I relaxed into the environment, I started to hear the sounds of the juvenile squirrels playing, calling each other, swinging on the diseased ash twigs which broke under their weight. The birdsong became part of the background, reducing in pitch and relaxing in timbre.

The next day, I awoke with the sun, having spent the night under the stars in the hammock. Then I heard the sounds of building work in the distance. Bristol has been undergoing a period of intense growth over the last year or two. Planning permission seems to get granted for almost every project, and why should that have been any different out here on the perimeter? A local once told me, 'They chopped down a whole row of trees — if they don't like trees, why live next to a forest?' Why indeed.

Despite the building work, after almost two days of being surrounded by trees, I started to feel a little different, a buzz about my body, like knots were untying. Like I'd had an acupuncture session or a good massage, or done a marathon session of t'ai chi.

By the third day, I was feeling even better. I watched a couple of ravens high up in the trees above my head. They had got closer and closer to my camp over the last few days as I'd become part of the scenery. I watched as they both took off at exactly the same time, flapping their wings in perfect unison, in harmony with their surroundings. I felt the same. A shift in my state of mind; something primal, slower.

One of the hallucinations I got while on *Amanita muscaria* (fly agaric mushrooms) was that the forest was flowing like a river, the browns and reds of the leaf litter bobbing up and down like waves. As I focused on it, it would start to flow into me — connecting me to the woodland and everything in it. That feeling came over me again, this time without the need for a mushroom. I felt a calm sense of oneness with my surroundings. Heard the buzz of insects, and squirrels chasing each other, high on hazelnuts (don't ask — it's a squirrel thing). It had been wet for the last few weeks and the forest had filled with a light mist as it warmed. It looked like it was full of thin will-o'-the-wisps,[19] magically dancing, like a blessing.

Over the last two decades that I've been working as a writer, I have taken moments when I disengage from the digital world. Often when crisis is looming, when anxiety is rising. I feel infinitely better for doing so. There are a number of studies to back this up; positive correlations have been found between mobile phone use and depression, anxiety, impulsivity, and poor sleep.[20] Newer technologies don't fare well, either; emerging research is suggesting that AI will add to the barrage of techno stresses we find ourselves subjected to.[21]

I can't help but feel old and nostalgic. Mine was the last generation that really enjoyed the freedoms of being able to make a fool of yourself without being filmed, and going to gigs without having to look through a thousand screens. I can remember a time when kids' TV lasted for a few hours a day, before 24-hour news and home computers, when a phone had a dial and was attached to a wall in a draughty hallway — that was, if you were *lucky* enough to afford a phone. It wasn't that we had to disengage from the digital world to feel more at ease with ourselves; it simply wasn't there.

Since then, the world has gone digital but, as I discussed in Chapter Two, I'm one of the 8 per cent of the country that doesn't have a smartphone. Life without a smartphone does present a few challenges. When my son started school, a WhatsApp group sprang up, and all the parents joined except for us. (Emma doesn't have a smartphone, either.) A whip-round happened for a Christmas gift for the teacher, a fistful of cycling vouchers. It was announced that 'all the families contributed but one'. Then questions came from my son: 'Daddy, are we poor?' I guess the assumption was that not having a smartphone, or a car, couldn't have been a choice.

Still, most of the time it's fine. I print off train tickets, I use *old-school* maps, I call people up or text to arrange meet-ups. I use social media on a web browser but only for short bursts, as I block myself using an app called Cold Turkey and am slowly deleting all my accounts. In other words, I live in the 1990s, and it's maybe more fun now than it was then, as I'm sober enough to enjoy it. Though, before this trip, I had been online more than usual, often googling symptoms Khloe was experiencing. Perhaps that was one of the reasons my mind was so frantic.

Away from all digital and family distractions, I started to notice many different things. I walked around the forest and pondered a line of web dangling in front of me. In it, a twig with two types of lichen on it was caught. I worried that the lichen would not be able to spread from there and wondered what I could do to help.

I felt distinctly odd that day, overwhelmed with empathy and emotion, similar to when my children were born, or before that when I used to take Ecstasy in my early twenties. A part of me worried that I was going a little bonkers, that a mixture of the microdosing and the utiseta had unhinged part of my brain. I need not have worried; on my return, I found the work of Rachel and Stephen Kaplan, a husband-and-wife team who developed a theory known as Attention Restoration Theory.[22] They helped to explain something of what I was feeling.

The Kaplans' research suggests that people who live in urban areas have constant demands on their attention. We walk along pre-designated paths, we read street signs (or Google Maps), we have to be aware of traffic — doubly so if we have children with us — and often we are focused on a task, an end goal — going to the shop for bread, for example. The same could be said of an artificial environment on a screen, such as a video game or app. This continual forced focus can lead to directed attention fatigue,[23] or the inability to carry out tasks that require our attention.

Learning this was a bit of a penny-dropping moment for me. What they described was what I'd call burnout, and I was certainly feeling it. The more time I spent on focused activity, be it work, caring for a child, or housework, the more likely I was to feel burned out. If I spent my whole time working, I became worse at what I was actually doing.

Directed attention fatigue can also lead to a host of other symptoms, such as increased aggression, feelings of unpleasantness, irritability, confusion, forgetfulness, acting out of character, inability to plan, and misperception of social cues;[24] it can also increase our stress levels. In short, if you are being a moody git, you may need to go for a walk in the park. It doesn't seem that different to the conclusions that Olmsted was coming up with almost 200 years ago.

I wonder how different things would have been if parks and gardens had remained important to planning bodies. I think of the third of all people in the UK and the USA who suffer with high anxiety levels.[25,26] Is it worth it for developers to make a little more money?*

I thought about what had led me to these feelings of moderate depression. My son was now old enough to take himself into school; my usual routine of adding a minimum of a mile to my walk home after the school run, up through the cemetery, was now gone. I'd been hammering social media; when I do that, my downtime becomes devoted either to thinking about what to put on my profile, scrolling or, at a push, thinking about what to write. I couldn't concentrate on anything, and I was starting to resort to magical thinking again. I thought about how much, or little, I'd been getting out since my utiseta. This was Nature Therapy 101, and I'd been failing.

I thought about all the other times in my life when I'd found myself acting out of character. Times when I wish I'd acted cooler and calmer — instead of starting a long feud with the neighbour who hates my foliage and has been known to dig up my bushes, maybe I didn't have to shout

---

* I don't like using the term 'developers' to mean property developer. A developer should be someone who aids growth or strengthens people; property developers often take something away from people.

at him. Considering I can see him from my window on a daily basis, it wasn't the best move. I thought about when I lived in Nottingham in a room that faced a brick wall, and worked on an industrial estate. How depressed I was. How my mood had always improved when I worked near trees or had an allotment.

Once, I worked for a bit on a cruise ship. It was a fairly long trip, 15 nights, most of them at sea. One afternoon, when the ship had been at sea for three days, and I was feeling particularly stir-crazy, I took a stroll to the back of the ship and stood staring out to sea in search of something real, anything. Without a connection to the outdoors or any greenery, my smoke hole was shut and I felt low — very low.

I could have tried circling the AstroTurfed deck again — but that made me feel worse somehow, like a trapped animal. The sea there was totally barren, devoid of all aquatic and avian life. The occasional oil tanker or cargo ship in the distance seemed to intensify this feeling. I tried looking up, but the sky was one big dirty-grey cloud. There were no seabirds following the boat, no dolphins, porpoises or whales; in fact, I never saw any fish or, for that matter, life in the water at all. We were nearing Africa, having just left the Canaries, and I wanted to see a life that wasn't human: a plant, an animal, even an insect. With the ship being sprayed daily, even the bacteria didn't stand a chance. I can remember marvelling at a single clothes moth that was jauntily flying around our room. But this eventually had to be killed to keep my cabin mate from flipping out.

It took me almost a month after we docked to stop feeling claustrophobic. I know many people love cruises and I don't decry them at all — some of my best friends even love to cruise. However, it turns out I really don't, and part of my mind stayed in that tiny cabin.

It being winter when we returned, it was hard to find much that was alive. My tonic? Eight hours with my fingers in soil, digging and preparing the ground on my allotment.

Carl Jung, the early psychologist and contemporary of Freud, would have highly approved. He believed that 'every human should have a plot of land so that their instincts can come alive again',[27] and with every shovelful of dirt, my instincts were coming alive again. An hour a day, across the winter months, digging, drinking tea, and sketching the occasional tree, was pure tonic.

The natural world isn't just something I love — it turns out to be something I need, something we all need. It helps me regulate my emotions and might perhaps help to alleviate much of the mental turmoil we suffer in the Western world. According to Harvard biologist E.O. Wilson, our brains developed in the natural world, making us 'hard wired' to respond positively to it.[28] Our brains are just not suited to the hustle, bustle, and grey concrete, steel, and glass dystopia of the human-created world. It's no wonder these environments can tire and stress us out. What is most interesting is that brain scans back up the theories of Wilson, the Kaplans, and Olmsted. They demonstrate that when shown natural and tranquil images rather than images of roads, disparate brain regions communicate with each other more easily.

Usually, after shorter afternoon or all-day trips to a forest, I feel something of the woods on me as I walk or cycle home. That feeling starts to dissipate as I walk, and I become more 'city'. This longer period was different, though. When

I returned home, I still felt that I was actually part of the forest.

I started to notice just how many trees, shrubs, and plants there actually were across the city. It felt like the forest stretched far beyond its border on the edge of the river, just beyond the city centre. Like it spread all the way to my home. I managed to stay rather blissed out for quite some time. To help me retain this feeling, Emma bought me a small fern, and I put that next to where I worked. I slowly filled the house with as many plants as I could. Friends got wind of what I was doing and offered me their suckers and runners — I duly accepted.

This helped, but I needed more. I could feel my stress levels increasing again. I was also getting angry at the cars selfishly parked on pavements as we walked about pushing Khloe's wheelchair. The roads are cramped near us, but they have got worse since cars have increased in size. Maybe I'd be more tolerant if I were a driver; maybe I'd have been more tolerant if I was getting more greenery in my life. I thought about Olmsted and put up an A5 picture of a forest near my desk. This wasn't enough, and my cubbyhole just felt more and more claustrophobic.

Eventually, I moved my desk to the window, where I sit now and type. Our garden is on a steep hill; the back of it is at eye level. I overlook my (good) neighbour Levi's garden. Thankfully, he's left it to go wild. The hazel bush fans out in all directions, catching the light on its leaves; the sun is starting its descent into autumn. Just up from this vision is the hedge of hawthorn, rose, and hazel that I planted a few years ago in my own garden. It is now at shoulder height and is often frequented by robins, goldfinches, and coal tits.

I can feel a daydreamy state come over me as I watch them. I'm more relaxed, less anxious, and I feel that maybe I've been a nicer person for the week since I moved my desk. It's helping, but is it enough?

About eleven days ago, I decided to give up furniture, to see how my body would react. In a chat with lifestyle and movement expert Billy Morgan from Movementum, he told me that 'Chronic niggles aren't a sign we are getting older, but a sign you've spent too much time being sedentary ... we live life in captivity ... and so we aren't going to be as if we were in our natural environment.' I wanted to see if there was any truth in Billy's statement, to see if I could be closer to my wild self in my own home. I also wanted to increase the amount of activity I did in the day.

I gave up my bed and slept on the floor. I changed my working set-up, carrying my office chair out of the corner of my bedroom and down into the living room, inadvertently turning the living room into a playground for my son. I then alternated between the floor and a crudely cobbled-together standing desk made by resting my screen on top of a chest of drawers and putting the keyboard onto a pulled-out drawer. Changes were made in other rooms, too. We eat two meals a day as a family at the dinner table in the kitchen. I decided to sit on the floor and eat my dinner there on a cushion, with a simple stool as a table. In the living room, I stopped sitting on the sofa, favouring floor cushions and the futon. I also decided to give up sitting on anything artificial outside the home — no chairs in cafes, no seats on public transport.

Each one of these decisions helped to maximise how often I shifted position or how much effort I'd need to take to move from a seated to an upright position. I knew this was a far cry from the semi-nomadic or hunter-gatherer lifestyle of constant movement lived by my ancestors, but at least I wasn't just sitting in a chair, allowing my body to accumulate any excess calories and turn them into fat.[29] I decided to keep a journal to log just how quickly I bounced from fairly fit human to fully fit Superdad, but reality had other plans.

It took giving up furniture, or at least beds and chairs, for me to realise just how im*bed*ded in our culture it is; pull up a chair, and I'll let you know how we got there. Beds in some form or other have been with us for as long as we can measure, and the oldest known mattress, made with reeds and rushes and strewn with medicinal plants to deter pests, dates to over 77,000 years ago.[30] It would have been about 30 centimetres (12 inches) off the floor. A similar floor-level bed, made from a filled pit, was found at the Hinds Cave site in Texas.[31] It would appear that we didn't rise off the floor until 5,000 years ago, when the ancient Egyptians created the raised bed — a sensible invention when you've rodents and snakes scurrying about.[32]

It's hard to pinpoint exactly where chairs really started but, according to architect and author Witold Rybczynski, the first historical record of a chair comes not from a written record but from a sculpted one: a flute player,[33] who may have once played to other ancient Greeks from his Aegean island home around 5,000 years ago.[34] The next move away from natural sitting came with the Egyptians. As is the case now, the elite started to ruin things for the rest of us, and their insistence on chairs with backs, rather than stools, started the trend that has infected much of the Western world.

So, then, that was my challenge: to live like humans did over 5,000 years ago, before the raised bed and the chair. The challenge of sleeping on the floor was the most difficult. I'm sure I've mentioned it before, but our house is not the biggest, and most of it is taken up by books and cooking equipment. In our bedroom, every square inch is utilised; my desk sits in the corner of the room with bookshelves above it. My office chair is sandwiched between a chest of drawers and the bed, with a bookshelf behind it. We've a double bed, but it only fits if it's rammed up next to the wall, leaving a small walkway that separates it from another two shelves: a wardrobe made from two exposed rails with another bookshelf, a chest of drawers, and our washing basket beneath it. This left me little room to sleep on the floor.

I squeezed a camping roll mat into the walkway and started to use that as my 'bed'. Note that I said I squeezed the camping roll mat into the walkway; needless to say, the first night I felt like I was stepping into a coffin. By the third night, I realised I'd got carpet burns from the side of the divan bed.

'Daddy, your job is too hard,' my daughter informed me after I complained that I was feeling a little tired. I was exhausted, in fact. Aching in places that I didn't think had ached for at least a decade. After only three days, I was ready to throw in the towel. Why would anyone choose to live like this?

I decided to move the roll mat into the living room, placing it on top of the futon — luxury. However, did I mention that we've all sorts of animals running in and out of the garden: badgers, hedgehogs, foxes, voles, and then a whole bunch of birds? One of them — I've still not narrowed down which — snuffles at the patio doors at first light, I discovered. Still, at least I was no longer living like Nosferatu the vampire.

This experiment was tough, really tough. Tougher than eating wild food (which I enjoyed), fasting (which I did not, but was at least only for 24 hours), naked camping, or anything else I had so far attempted in response to my call of the wild. According to author and movement expert Katy Bowman in her book *Rethink Your Position*,[35] our cells will adapt and 'fail to develop the strength and mobility needed to minimise and withstand the pressures of our own bodyweight'. She states that this is true not just of chairs and beds, but of pillows and shoes. Bowman recommends that we train ourselves little by little, just as we would if we were training to run a marathon. This allows the body to readapt to a more natural posture. I didn't train myself gradually like this, thinking that I'd be okay, and I now regretted it.

When I sat back — or crouched down — and thought about it, I'd struggled with suppleness for many years. I don't think I've touched my toes since childhood, and I gave up Buddhism because I couldn't sit cross-legged or sit unsupported with a straight back for long enough. The pain was too distracting for me to get any kind of enlightenment. I'm as supple as a plank of wood.

I found it particularly hard to adopt a position that suited me to work without a chair. I tried sitting on the floor with a laptop, but my back started to ache very quickly. I tried sitting on a floor cushion and elevated the laptop, thinking that would help — it didn't. I then tried standing, and that was okay for a bit, but it soon got exhausting, plus the wind was taken out of my sails a little after reading that standing desks come with their own issues, including increased lower back problems![36]

I decided that a little workaround was in order. What alternatives were there? Vaguely remembering a documentary I'd seen about Indigenous people all sitting in a hammock, I surmised that this *bed* might be ancient enough to be the solution. Besides, the act of getting in and out of a hammock prompted more movement than getting in and out of a chair or bed — that was enough for me. But had they really been around long enough for me to justify using one? I studied the literature. Turns out that the Indigenous folks of the Americas pre-colonisation had several types of hammock. The Ipurina, of the Amazon basin, used three long strips of bark, which they tied up at both ends. The Timbira and Xerénte used leaves that interlocked.[37] There were plenty more examples across the Americas. I also found reference to a medieval hammock here in the UK,[38] a picture of a piece of cloth tied between two posts.

My back told me that this was plenty of evidence, and I quickly switched to sitting in a hammock, moving my screen around my bedroom/office as I found the optimum position — the unused bed a resting place for my monitor. I then started to sleep in the hammock and, though I'm sure that didn't help my back either, it was good to be back in the bedroom. There are times, especially when working on a book, when I suffer from middle-of-the-night insomnia. I wake up in need of the loo and then sit like a wide-eyed aye-aye for up to an hour or more. Thoughts race through my head, and I can't sleep until I quieten them. There was now a solution to hand — literally; I could extend a hand out of the hammock and leisurely push. This would gently rock the hammock and send me back off to sleep rather quickly. This set-up worked well for a few days, but into the third week my back started to really ache. After a while, I realised that I'm just not used to sitting without support for this long, nor am I used to sleeping in anything other than a bed. According to the *New Scientist*,[39] too much sitting may have reduced my natural range of motion due to a shortening of my hip and knee flexor muscles.

My experience is no different from that of around 60 per cent of the Western world,[40] who will, at some point in their lives, suffer from lower back pain. I'd read that obesity can dramatically increase back trouble.[41] A year or two before I wrote this book, I'd shifted about 18 kilograms (40 pounds) through a regime of hill walking and intermittently fasting for 13–16 hours a day, and, to keep it off, I cut out refined sugar completely from my diet. This all helped dramatically, and the back pain had become less and less frequent.

This time around, though, it wasn't just back pain, and it wasn't just that I was aching all over; I also felt depressed, and that was adding to the problem. The back pain wasn't the thing that was making me feel depressed, but the depression was giving me back pain. They fed each other like a co-dependent couple. I knew it wasn't because of my outsider status at home, although my family had all started throwing peas at me from their superior spots at the table. No, other than that one mealtime, we were actually feeling very close as a family — adversity does that.

Then, one morning, I had an epiphany. I'd been writing down my dreams and analysing them — it gave me insights into feelings and emotions I might have missed during the day. I had dreamed that I was a complete outsider, shunned by everyone I met. I ended up crying on the shoulder of a drag queen that I know — someone who is a total extrovert when working, but on a personal level is a complete introvert, shy and awkward, often inhabiting the perimeter of a party or gathering; also an outsider. In the dream, I was both the person being hugged and the hugger. I realised that I was becoming an outsider due to this experiment. The world sits on chairs. I knew that I was trying to accomplish something I could never accomplish too quickly. I couldn't hope to suddenly be much fitter in a week.

Furthermore, I'd taken away any kind of coping mechanism I might have had, alienating myself from every comfort. I'd robbed myself of all the things I enjoy doing in my city — grabbing a break, a read or a sketch, having a coffee when I'm out and about all involve sitting; so does going for a pint with a friend. I've always hated *standing* at the bar. I wondered if I could even allow myself to go for a shit, as my loo is the conventional Western style, which, if you think about it, is nothing more than a chair with a hole in it! My allotment and the local wild cemetery are both places I like to sit. I have my favourite benches in the cemetery, and on the allotment I sit in a chair for a cup of tea before I start work. I noticed that on the three occasions I automatically sat down without thinking — once on a chair I thought about buying in a shop, and twice in the morning — it was quickly followed by a feeling of pleasure, a dopamine hit, a sign of a pleasurable and entrenched habit.[42] I didn't realise this before, but I'm a chair addict. I've lived like this for almost five decades, and it now hurts my back if I try anything other than sitting on a chair with a back. I am like much of the Western world: my body has grown to favour the chair to such an extent that it's almost impossible to live without it. In fact, I found it quite lonely and awkward.

Think about your life: are you a habitual chair user, too? The whole of Western culture sits on chairs; they are the exemplars of our society — a society addicted to and, ultimately, damaged by comfort. We force chair dependence on ourselves almost as soon as we are born. Think about it: hospital-born kids are not allowed to leave the hospital without a car seat; it's hospital policy across the Western world. If you try to break this policy and get on a bus or into a car without a car seat, in the UK at least, you'd be breaking the law.[43] Before you shout, 'What about home births?', there simply aren't many; over the last six decades there has been a definite shift away from the practice, with only 1–2.9 per cent of births now at home. Perhaps you could walk with your bundle of joy swaddled in a sling; however, the average distance from a maternity hospital to a home is about seven miles (11.3 kilometres) — a distance that's walkable but perhaps not that appealing to someone who's just given birth. It's a perfect storm that means the first moments of human life are spent sitting in a seat.

As your child grows, so do the products on offer, restricting natural strengthening exercises and ignoring how kids might naturally want to sit,[44] creating the groundwork for future back problems. We were guilty of this and bought a bouncy chair for sitting in the living room, a high chair for the dinner table, and a pushchair to transport our kids around. We'd pick them up off the floor, where they naturally wanted to sit, and plonk them down in these expensive items of transitory furniture.

School starts in reception year with children sitting on the floor — so far, so good — but the next year they have a mixture of floor and chairs. This is slowly phased out as they age, and by the time they are eight they are forced to sit on chairs for the whole school day. I remember being reprimanded for bad behaviour when I leaned forward in my school chair, squatting, perhaps instinctively trying to correct my posture to something more natural. After all, the squat is the position favoured by people in South-East Asia, Africa, and Latin America.[45] Arguably, this might be the most natural position for humans to sit in, as it is how our nearest relative, the chimpanzee, chooses to sit.

But does living without a chair make that much difference to posture, strength, and our overall health? Perhaps it doesn't matter that I've a back that is as strong as a cup of overly milky tea made with third-hand Happy Shopper tea leaves. I mean, apart from the odd niggle, I can live with it, can't I? It seems not, as evidence points to chair dependency leading to an early death. One study suggests that sitting for over six hours of leisure time a day meant an increased mortality rate of 37 per cent for women and 17 per cent for men.[46] But I moved a lot, or at least I felt like I did, even in a chair. Didn't I?

I decided to find out and took a time-lapse film of myself sitting in a hammock and sitting in a chair in order to look for differences. I was hoping to simply count the number of times I moved in a hammock,[47] and the number of times I moved in a chair.[48] A crude test, and not without its faults — the main one being that my behaviour was undoubtedly influenced by the outcome I wanted. However, the results were so stark that I believe them to be useful. In the hammock, I moved constantly; in the chair, I stayed totally stationary. I started to think that I had this down: I visualised myself at 80 years old, nimbly getting in and out of my hammock as I went about my working day.

My 80-year-old self would have avoided all the health issues associated with my chair sitting, such as lower back pain,[49] cardio metabolic diseases like diabetes and heart trouble,[50] early muscle fatigue, decreased muscle elasticity, blood clots, and sleep apnoea.[51] I also felt like I'd found a magic bullet allowing me to work as an author, a job that necessitates a whole load of sitting, and still being able to reach the ripe old age of 80. In fact, I now started to picture myself at 100.

I was premature in my thinking. I started to notice a bit of a twinge in my back and in my knee. I kidded myself that I'd be fine. It was nothing to worry about. The back pain started in the hammock one evening, and it kept waking me up. It was sharp and acute. I'd just slept a little wrongly, I reassured myself — nothing to worry about. Then the knee pain started while I was squatting to talk to Khloe on the bus. I felt a heat coming from my joint; it was shouting at me to sit, but I was determined to live to 100 and wasn't listening. I can be quite stubborn if I make a rule — single-minded, you might say — and I'd made a rule for myself that I wouldn't even sit on a bus or train. Cars were okay, because I didn't have much choice. So, every journey I took, I'd squat or stand next to Khloe — even though there were plenty of spare seats. I stood on the train across town, too.

What's more, my squatting on cushions was starting to niggle as well. This body, my body, is not used to doing things differently, and it had been trying to tell me so. The words of Katy Bowman were ringing in my ears: 'We train ourselves little by little just as we would if we were training to run a marathon.' I'd gone from couch to marathon, and now I was paying for it.

It was time to admit defeat. I decided to take stock, not to run into this blindly. That evening, I unclipped my hammock and brought my office chair back into my room. I made my bed, and I jumped in and slept. It was a bit overshadowed by feelings of failure, but it was nonetheless comfortable. The next day, I sat back in my office chair. It was like being reunited with an old friend. I'd been using this chair for about three years now and knew its quirks.

But over the next few days, I realised that some of the things had stuck — the things that brought pleasure. Every Tuesday we have started to have tacos. I know, I know, it's not the wildest of meals, but it's easy and a bit fun. It's a kind of indoor picnic, laying out all the food on our rug and choosing our own fillings. The new layout of floor cushions and futon mean we are all at the same level and closer, all of us naturally shunning the sofa. We also seem to arrange ourselves in a circle. There is a different feeling to this mealtime, a closeness, and conversation is subtly different than at the dinner table. There isn't the battle against reading at the table, and there are more smiles. There is also very little pea-throwing. The success has led to Pizza Friday. They are both mealtimes we all look forward to. It also means that Khloe doesn't have to rely on us to lift her up on to a chair. As I sat at this level, I pondered what parliament might look like if they met on the floor instead of in their gladiatorial-style set-up, sitting across from the enemy in hierarchical rows — the most powerful at the bottom for all to see, backed up by their tribe of warring allies behind them. A sure-fire set-up for confrontation.

Our own confrontations can happen at night as I corral the kids upstairs for a bedtime story. But our new set-up seemed to help. The kids enjoyed the hammock in the bedroom, too, and it was soon re-clipped not for me to work from, but as a perch for reading both to the kids and to myself. I find myself getting a lot of pleasure from the fact that I can gently swing in the hammock while reading. I may be sitting in my office chair again, but the other chairs are being shunned. I hope that it helps to set in motion a lifestyle choice that will keep my kids jumping in and out of hammocks right up into their eighties and nineties.

Over a year since I started writing this chapter, I still have a hammock in the bedroom and two in the garden. I sit in them whenever I get the chance, and the kids, and their friends, still love them. In fact, every night one of them will sit in the hammock while I sit on the bed reading to them. It's created a very comfortable and uncluttered space for us all to enjoy in my library, bedroom, and office.

The futon has remained in the living room, and it continues to be my seat of choice. Sometimes, I find myself wanting to sit on the floor in the kitchen, or I hop up and sit on the units. I'm no longer uncomfortable without a backrest. Most importantly, though, I've not had any back trouble in over a year, despite having prolonged periods of sitting while I write. My knees are stronger and more resilient, too. Last week, my now 11-year-old son jumped on my back as I was walking downstairs. I was taking a step down as he did it; I had to quickly compensate for the extra weight and awkwardly took a step down on to the next stair, jarring my knee as I did so (yes, there was swearing; no, it wasn't pretty). It was painful, very painful. I expected the healing process to take some time and worried I'd be out of action. I wasn't — it healed in a day or two.

I've also noticed that a little bit of discomfort bothers me much less than it did. That I can camp again, something I thought I'd grown out of. Overall, I feel like I've been given an extra little magic pill of health. That the small changes I've implemented have made a difference. Lifestyle coaches might advocate a completely new regime, but these little extra tweaks have made a difference to me, giving me a better quality of life as I head into the next stage.

On top of that, I'm now a lot more mindful of the time I spend indoors. I'm slowly moving myself outdoors as much as I can. My desk remains facing the window, and I go out for walks even in the December gloom. The thought of going out always puts a smile on my face. When I'm distracted now, it is by the many birds that visit the garden or fly overhead — even in the winter we have ravens, blackbirds, robins, and goldfinches all over the place in my wild garden.

As I think back on all the houses and flats I've lived in — places sometimes without gardens, bedrooms without windows, or views out onto treeless roads, brick walls or main roads with nothing but the top deck of the bus looking back — I think of how, if there is a mistake in a recipe that we're following in a book, we blame ourselves for getting it wrong before we blame the book. It feels the same with living spaces: that, fundamentally, our culture and our man-made environment are at fault, and we are blaming ourselves for our natural reactions to it. Perhaps town planners and property developers are more to blame for the rising rates of anxiety and depression than we are as individuals. Perhaps some of their profits need to be syphoned back into the system to pay for the harm they have caused.

When I'm not working, I'm out all the time, but when I am working, I try to have a walk and sit out somewhere natural every day, even if it is just to have a cup of tea in the hammock in the back garden. I also break up my day with slightly longer walks to the nearby park and cemetery. I've noticed I'm more productive when I get to do this, less distractible. The social media block really does help; it gives me back my time. I think it gives me the ability to earn more, too, as away from it my mind is sharper and more focused when it needs to be, and calmer when it doesn't. I can ponder more things, slowly come to solutions rather than making snap decisions that turn out to be the worst choice possible. I've also started to notice that I like to sit and do nothing but look out at the greenery of the garden.

I get the bus out to the Mendips and go for a walk at least once a week. I've started to write more in notepads while sitting under trees or next to rivers, drafting essays or writing poetry. I'm currently trying to work out if I can move my writing practice offline. If I could write the first draft of a book in pen and maybe type it up with my voice, while sitting in a hammock. It feels like the right way to live. I just wish you could all find a way to have the same.

NEW WILD YOUR SHELTER

If you have a desk job, consider moving your desk so that it faces out towards some greenery; rearrange the office if you have to. Quote from this chapter if you need to convince a boss of this move; be sure to mention the decrease in sick days caused by stress.

Before you switch all your furniture for floor furniture, try sitting on the floor using the sofa as a backrest for one evening a week. Slowly increase this as your body gets used to the change. As you get stronger, switch to a floor cushion and/or just the floor.

Introduce floor picnics once a week.

Buy, or make, a hammock and attach it to two load-bearing walls inside your house. Try using this as an office chair. If you have the space, try introducing one to the garden, too. A hammock under a tree is the ideal, as there is no better spot than looking up into its branches.

Introduce outdoor working whenever possible.

Explore your local area. Find the wildest areas possible and try to incorporate these places into your daily routine — perhaps taking a slightly longer walk to get your shopping, or to the bus stop.

Leave your mobile phone at home for at least two hours once a week and reflect on how it makes you feel.

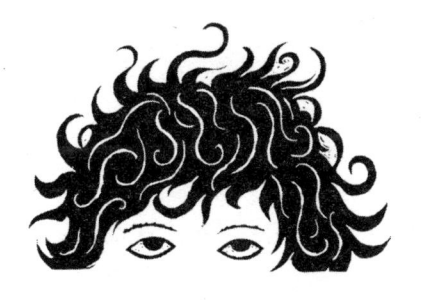

CHAPTER FOUR

Bodies

'Soap and education are not as sudden as a massacre, but they are more deadly in the long run'

MARK TWAIN, 1875

Imagine working somewhere you have to take a lift every morning. You are 60 storeys up, so stairs are not an option. Imagine that there are always two identical lifts to choose from: Lift A and Lift B. Both will get you where you need to be at the same time. The only difference is that the elevator operator in Lift A doesn't use soap or cleaning products, and the one in Lift B uses a plethora of soaps, detergents, scents, and creams. Also imagine that the lifts are rather troublesome and, despite getting you to your floor, they are very slow — you are going to spend a long time in that lift with the elevator operator. Which do you choose?

You may instinctively choose Lift B; after all, the average

time humans spend on grooming adds up to 1.1 hours a day,[1] almost four times the amount of time that we, as a species, spend looking after children. You might think that Lift A will be smelly and B far more pleasant — because who wants to smell any kind of body odour? However, choosing Lift A could help to reduce your anxiety levels.[2] If you choose Lift B and you are asthmatic, it could be the last lift ride you ever take. Around one-third of us are irritated by artificial scents,[3] and by 'irritated' I really mean having allergic reactions, which can range from a runny nose and streaming eyes to coughs and even asthma attacks.

I'm sensitive to many smells. I have to swap carriages on trains, vent hotel rooms or pull the batteries out of air fresheners. On more than one occasion, I've had to leave a room if someone has been wearing too much scented deodorant or perfume, or has washed their hair with a potent shampoo. My family are sensitive, too, and with two asthmatics at home, we have to be careful. A well-meant bag full of children's clothes once given to us had to be fumigated before they were used, so strong was the scent of laundry soap. Three of us had streaming noses and eyes. For me, it can trigger sinusitis, which can be so severe that I wind up in bed for a day or two.

Interestingly, these strong reactions might be protecting us. Links are now being made between our overuse of cosmetics and an increase in allergies. A few years ago, a Japanese company had to withdraw some facial soap that contained hydrolysed wheat protein,[4] after more than 500 people with no history of food allergies claimed to have had an allergic reaction to it. In fact, in around 70 people it was so severe that they passed out. Scented products might also be adding to the problem of pollution in our towns and cities. In a recent study, emissions from our deodorants now rival those of transport.[5]

The cosmetics industry is one that has grown enormously in recent years. My parents, both born just after 1945, take great joy in reminiscing about a time when the bathroom was a tin bath in front of the fire, and the toilet was a cold, spider-ridden outhouse with newspaper on a bit of string where the toilet roll would be now. For night-time calls of nature, there was a chamber pot, or *guzunder*. This was a kind of potty for grown-ups that goes under (*guzunder*) the bed. There was still a bit of a hangover from this time when I was a child and we visited elderly relatives; my brother and I used to find it hilarious if we were given an adult potty to see us through the night.

Now that I'm a parent, I find I suffer from the same misty-eyed moments. The guzunder, tin bath, and outdoor toilets had all but disappeared by the 1970s and 1980s, but compared to now, the range of cosmetics and bathroom facilities was much smaller. We had no on-demand hot water and had to wait for a single bath's worth to share, drawing straws for who'd go first. There was no shower other than an attachment that kept falling off the taps. Most of all, there was a distinct lack of products. Hair conditioner didn't arrive in our house until the nineties; we didn't all have our own different kinds of toothpaste, as my kids do; my dad's razors were single-bladed Bic ones that *glided* over your skin like a drunken elephant; soap came in a bar and had one smell, and there was no liquid soap. We did have bubble bath but no bath salts, bath bombs or body scrubs. Most of all, though, I can remember that deodorant was only ever worn by women. This was a time when synthetic fabrics were still all the rage, and my overriding childhood memory of my parents' generation is that — close up, at least — the men smelled! I don't remember it being a bad thing; they just smelled like grown-ups. I feel like my kids' generation is sometimes robbed of that comforting smell. It was the smell of a piggyback ride, a friendly wrestling match, the smell of fathers.

Ridding ourselves of these nostalgic odours, we might be throwing the bacteria out with the bathwater. Life expectancy in Europe and the USA is now declining,[6,7] and, in a phone conversation with Dr George Moncrieff, a leading UK dermatologist and former chair of the Dermatology Council for England, he stated that 'we are in very real danger of developing serious antibiotic resistance, where bacteria will adapt to no longer be affected by antibiotics, and diseases that used to be curable — like tuberculosis, which in the 1800s used to kill 25 per cent of the European population — will start killing us again'. Although this resistance has been attributed to our overconsumption of antibiotics and their use in livestock, fingers are also starting to be pointed at our overuse of soap and detergents. It turns out that it might be a bad idea to undo millions of years of coexistence with the bacteria that once thrived on our skin and the comforting, familiar smells they help to produce.

Our skin is nothing short of amazing. It doesn't just sit there on top of tissue and muscle, not doing much; it is active, dynamic, and the largest organ in the body. It is our first line of defence against viruses and other pathogens, acting as a primary barrier. It also acts as an interface with the outside world and other humans.[8] Goosebumps, for example — the little pinprick bumps on your skin that are accompanied by hairs standing on end — are your skin's natural response to being cold or having heightened emotions. This action was much more useful when we had more hair, though. Consider a cat for a second: when she leaves the house and it's cold, having her hairs stand on end not only makes her look bigger and therefore more menacing to other cats but also traps warm air, helping to keep her insulated.

Sadly, I found it impossible to locate any research to back up my theory that anyone who excessively shaves their body hair is colder than those who don't. Although, reassuringly, some studies are starting to suggest another reason for getting goosebumps is that longer periods of cold and the subsequent goosebumps might even help to stimulate hair growth.[9] As bills rise and my hairline retreats, turning off the heating is starting to look more appealing.

Our skin's reactions might do more than help our hair grow. Skin sends out other signals, too, turning ashen when we are sick and therefore signalling the need for help or quarantine. We can turn red to signal embarrassment, shame, and guilt. If you are someone who goes red at the drop of a hat, be reassured: this might be a very handy evolutionary adaptation. It's considered that the redder we go, the more likely we are to be forgiven by others for our crime or misdemeanour.[10]

I wonder if those of you who thought you'd prefer to travel in the scented lift might actually do something different in reality, especially if you are single, as your skin does one more interesting thing: it can attract a mate. We signal arousal to each other with increased activity in our sweat glands.[11]

Our sweat glands, or apocrine glands, secrete proteins and lipids into our hair follicles, which in turn travel up onto the skin. This is food for the bacteria that live in our armpits and groin, and it is their waste products that can cause body odour. This odour can attract a mate or signal danger, part of the reason why sweat might be smellier when we are aroused or stressed. Shaving our groin or under our arms, or using deodorant, while reducing odour, can decrease the signals we are sending out. When I was single, I wonder if I ever considered that the products I was using to make myself more attractive could actually be having the opposite effect.

Despite how wonderful our skin is naturally, billions of pounds of advertising has convinced us that we need to manage it with creams, chemicals, deodorants, and detergents. We have been conditioned to believe that 100 years of product development is superior to the fine-tuning of millions of years of evolution. It's like saying a toddler with an iPad can create original works of literature to rival Shakespeare, Flora Nwapa, Laozi, Chaucer, Maya Angelou, and James Baldwin all rolled together.

We throw money at making our skin artificially shine, but the real cost could be far greater. The most common problem with our skin is eczema. Only 2–3 per cent of the post-war generation suffered from it, and it was even considered an affliction of the elite. Many families in the UK lived in cramped conditions and worked long hours; children were ushered out of the house to play in order for housewives to be able to keep house. I'm not saying this was a good set-up, for any of those involved, but what I am saying is that the children of my grandparents' generation had to be rich in order to have the time and space to want to be indoors.

Things have changed dramatically: most kids will now spend less time outdoors than a prison inmate,[12] and around 30 per cent of children under the age of 15 suffer from atopic eczema. There is a theory that sun exposure prevented eczema due to increased rates of vitamin D, and that subsequent lack of outdoor play helped to trigger higher rates.[13] This has been compounded by our use of cosmetics on the skin, which remove the natural oils that also keep eczema in check.[14] With indoor activities and bathrooms now the norm, and trillions of dollars spent yearly on cosmetics, are we all now the elite?[15] And are we paying the price for it?

It is thought that our ancestors would have used sand and mud as occasional exfoliants,[16] and perhaps a stone to scrape it all off,[17] but that was it. It wasn't until the ancient Babylonians started burning the plant soapwort and mixing it with water to wash that we first started to use a form of soap.[18] Originally, it wasn't used to wash with daily; instead, people used the mix to do the dishes, wash their clothes and, on occasion, treat skin diseases.

After that, the history of soap-making is a bit muddy, but the most interesting tale takes us to Mount Sapo, near Rome, about 3,000 years ago. This was a place of animal sacrifice, and the animals would afterwards be burned. The fat from the animals would mix with the potash of the fire, turning it into a slippery clay which ran down the slopes like lava. It was soon discovered that this 'clay of Sapo' could be used to wash clothes. The practice took a while to catch on around the globe, with sporadic use throughout different civilisations. In fact, during the Middle Ages, some factions of the Christian Church in Europe even sought to ban it, for fear of our succumbing to sin by exposing ourselves to too much flesh. Back then, cleanliness was next to devilishness.

The business of soap-making started to gather pace by the mid-19th century, when the process became industrialised. With money to earn, attitudes needed to be changed. This was a time when disease and death would come knocking at most people's doors, and when microscopic germ theory was (correctly) linking the fecal–oral route with cholera. In this climate of fear, a London-based dermatologist named Erasmus Wilson published *Healthy Skin* (1845), a publication that linked the moral cleanliness of workers with the physical cleanliness of their skin and households,[19] his words helping to launch the iconic advertising campaign for Pears soap. Keeping the skin clear of the sweat, dirt, and filth of disease-ridden Victorian Britain set a rather solid stage for the future of the skincare industry and the mysophobic world which prevails to this day.

The truth is, we don't need all these products to keep our skin functioning and healthy. People such as journalist, author, and doctor James Hamlin are part of a growing army who are finding out just how little we need to use soap.[20] He describes cases of friends who gave up using soap and found their acne cleared up. Moncrieff told me that not using detergents on the body often helps eczema sufferers. It makes sense: anything that can help the diversity of our microbiota, the ecosystem that is our microbiome, helps our health. Medical microbiologist Dries Budding agrees.

He believes that our bodies are similar to a forest or even the ocean — the more varied the population living in it, the healthier it is. Budding suggests that you are more likely to suffer from athlete's foot and other fungal infections the more you use soap.

In other words, capitalism is creating a problem and selling us the solution. Yet, we are all so complicit in this that we have started to think that anyone who doesn't smell like a duty-free shop in an airport is somehow dirty, and we'd refuse to get in a lift with them.

Still, people like Hamlin have broken the trend, and he has gone without soap, other than on his hands, for the last six years. He suggests that as he used less, he started to need less. I thought I'd give it a go, first on my hair — with mixed results.

The benefits of looking good in front of other human beings are clear: it doesn't just attract a mate but can secure us a better job,[21] and even help to decrease a prison sentence.[22] Cosmetic companies are fully aware of this, and it helps them to market a host of products that can trigger fears of unattractiveness.

Campaigns in the UK and Europe often focus on how damaged and lifeless hair can be revitalised or how greasy hair can be cured, while — currently, at least — the US focuses on how much stronger a person you can be when using a certain shampoo.[23] My favourite fear-triggering campaign comes from Myanmar and gives the suggestion that dandruff can cause everyone at a party to shun you like the flaky-scalped social pariah you are.[24]

These advertisers are playing on real fears of being seen as dirty, limp-haired or even flaky-scalped, which began in the 1970s, a time when haircare products really started to take off. One swish of her perfect hair and Farrah Fawcett had us all too keen to believe that shampoo was the only route to being equally fabulous-looking. Soon, much of the world was hooked on shampoo. We quickly went from using soap on our hair around once a month to using shampoo almost every day.

Being born in the 1970s, I distinctly remember only getting my hair washed once every two weeks. As I grew into a teenager and found myself in charge of my own hair, insecurity kicked in, and I upped my game considerably. By the time I was 25 and working in an office, each morning saw me alternating washing my hair with shaving; I never had time to do both on the same day. Every other day I'd have greasy-looking hair, and I'd tie it up or cover it in talc to try to disguise it. Mostly, though, I just felt very self-conscious about it. The advertising campaigns had done their damage.

Around ten years ago, my partner, Emma, suggested I try Aleppo soap, a Castile soap made using just olive oil, lye, and laurel oil, instead of shampoo; she'd been to Syria (pre-2011 outbreak of conflict), come back with a few bars, and was emphatic about how good they left her hair feeling. I was sceptical at first; I mean, soap is meant to wash our skin, not our hair. But she has this way of repeating things that she thinks will benefit me until my stubbornness subsides, so after my initial resistance I tried it.

I'm not sure why I was so resistant to this; after all, I had been looking for an alternative since I'd heard that some of the chemicals found in shampoo are thought to increase the risk of certain cancers,[25] disrupt our brain development,[26] and interfere with our hormones.[27] Suffering from occasional hypochondria, I wanted rid. Further studies suggest that these risks might turn out to be unfounded and are low, so I shouldn't worry. However, that might be beside the point; they may be okay individually, but together they add to the toxic cocktail of products we can find in our homes, and that could prove a problem. Lab experiments find it hard to test this, as they often only replicate being exposed to one chemical at a time.[28]

Over the next three years, I used just soap on my hair. I noticed two things. Firstly, my hair didn't get so greasy, and so I didn't need to wash it nearly as much. Secondly, I started to really notice the synthetic smell of freshly shampooed hair when out in the park or woods. It still bothers me a little, as it sits in the air unnaturally for longer than many other scents, and walking in the slipstream of it always makes my nose twitch.

I was happy with my soap-twice-a-week routine, as was Emma with her thick, dark, beautiful hair. Then I spoke to a mum in the local play park. She told me how she didn't wash her kid's hair at all, as he reacted to anything she put on it. So one morning, without researching it first, I stopped using anything in my hair. I'd just had my hair cut rather short and felt that it would be the easiest time to dive in.

Within a week, my fine, mousey-coloured hair developed a rather wayward personality, sticking up all over the place. But, crucially, no one said, 'Your hair is greasy,' or even let their eyes linger for a moment or two longer than they should have on my scalp. After six weeks of nothing, not even water in my hair, I felt I'd cracked it.

Then I noticed a bad smell, like mice had got in. I checked the house for holes, cleaned under the cooker and fridge, put food on high shelves — all the things you do to protect against rodents. I thought that would be enough, but then I noticed the smell while out with friends. It was following me about. I was mortified. I got my kids to smell my hair, and they took great joy in telling me that, sure enough, I was the smell.

If I was honest, I had just jumped into this experiment without any prep — what was I expecting? I hadn't even been using water to rinse out the build-up of everything a city can throw at us. I had noticed a feeling of something on my scalp, but instead of doing something about it, I ignored it, thinking that tackling it would ruin the experiment. A very quick search later and I had a solution: bicarbonate of soda. I plastered on big dollops of the stuff. My hair felt wonderful — soft and clean and great — and what's more, the smell had gone.

That was the start of a spiral of events. A few weeks later, and I had the world's worst case of dandruff. Scales everywhere — the case for a return to shampoo was starting to strengthen. Then my face started to develop a red, itchy, unsightly rash. It soon spread across my face, and the itching was so unbearable it would keep me up at night. This lasted for about a month and, thinking it was something to do with giving up washing, I started to use soap on my face again. It didn't help. In desperation, I used various moisturisers and anti-fungal creams, which just seemed to make matters worse. I was back into the vicious cycle of cleanliness.

Turns out it was seborrhoeic dermatitis, the same condition that causes dandruff, and it had spread to my face. I had dandruff of the scalp *and* face. The smell had been the start of it, caused by a build-up of Malassezia yeast — a yeast that 100 per cent of us naturally have growing on us. But my body had decided this was a threat and was overproducing skin cells to try to combat it. It was made worse as I was stressing out about work and travelling to see my elderly parents during a pandemic.

To compound the issue, the medication I'm on to keep my autoimmune condition in check also means I'm more prone to things like fungal infections. Other risk factors included being in my forties — as I am — and cold weather — it was winter. I wondered if there should be another box that I could tick: idiot. Undeterred, I had a quick search around and found that the likely culprit was that the dandruff from my scalp had started to fall onto my face. I didn't feel any less unclean for knowing this. What it did make me realise was that my regime would have to take my medical condition into consideration, as well as my age and the season.

Then I found a technique that YouTubers were calling 'medieval combing'.[29] Essentially, you comb your hair backwards for around 30 minutes a day, and this helps to reduce dandruff and rids you of the fungus. I hoped it would also keep the dandruff from falling on my face. My GP agreed and suggested that products never cure seborrhoeic dermatitis; they only keep the symptoms at bay. She also recommended going out in the sun a little more. I realised I had got into a bad winter habit of only going out for around one hour a day.

I started to garden again, and this helped my stress levels. I also began brushing my hair backwards, not for 30 minutes a day — that was ridiculous — but just when the urge hit me. Sometimes in batches of five minutes multiple times a day, sometimes for longer; I suspect it probably added up to about 30 minutes, but I wasn't exact. Within two days, the seborrhoeic dermatitis had started to clear up and never got to the acute itchy stage again. Also, my hair started to look and feel great, and, what's more, the smell didn't return. Combing had become the new shampooing! After a while, I knew the signs of it returning. I'd shave my beard off, splash water on my face three times a day, and go out as much as possible — all of that helped.

Three years on and I'd forgotten about the combing. The dandruff returned, and I'm sad to report that I've returned to shampoo. I just got fed up with people staring at my scalp — or at least, I got fed up of thinking that people were. It's always worse in the winter months; in the summer I can return to no 'poo. I am envious of others who can practise this year-round. My friend Deepak says he hasn't washed his thick black hair for 24 years. He just massages it after wetting it in the shower. I never noticed, but he also admitted to not owning a comb. Lucky bastard!

However, I don't feel fully beaten. The New Wild Order process is ongoing and adapts with the circumstances and the individual, after all. I've since had apple cider vinegar (ACV) recommended for dandruff. I used a ratio of one-quarter of a 250-millilitre mug full of ACV to three-quarters warm water* and, after just one application, I've noticed a vast improvement; it's also given my thinning hair a little extra body. I'm not sure how often I'll need to use it, and I think I may also use it on my beard. I'm very happy to have found a bit of a natural solution after what

---

* Thank you, Molly Slight.

feels like a long voyage of discovery.

In comparison, giving up soap elsewhere was rather uneventful. There was no great smell, and I know my kids would have told me if there had been. I have to admit that one of my biggest worries was giving up soap on my armpits. So I got a crystal stone deodorant and started using it daily. Crystal stone is an alternative deodorant made of potassium alum, a natural mineral salt that occurs as an encrustation on rocks. It has been used in South Asia for centuries. Considering that the most common allergy to cosmetics is to deodorant,[30] this natural alternative seemed to be a worthwhile concession.[31]

Then I employed the sniff test: if I smelled bad, I'd use it. I noticed that I'd often smell worse if I'd been wearing synthetic fibres. Luckily, I wrote this bit when I first got my advance for this book, and so was in the position to shell out for a bunch of new pure-cotton and hemp shirts. Soon I noticed that I was saving on clothes washing, too; with my armpits able to breathe more easily, I could wear shirts for more than the one day, as I had been doing. Hemp was particularly good and lasted for up to four days without the need for a spin. Other adopters of the soap-on-hands-only regime have noted that they got smellier the more stressed they were and so have to adjust their regime accordingly.

Four years later, and I still only wash with soap under my arms and sometimes on my head, a habit that looks set to continue for life. To admit this to the book-buying public still feels like I've broken a massive taboo. I feel like the person in Lift A, shunned for breaking a cultural norm set in motion by cholera-ridden London. Considering the budget for convincing people not to use products will always be 100 per cent less than the budget for making them use products, I may be riding alone in a lift for some time yet.

I wondered what other products we are led to believe we need: aftershave, a bigger car — or a car, full stop — bigger, more powerful mobile phones, and faster broadband. I thought about how not having a smartphone has become a statement rather than what feels like the right choice for my own mental health. 'Your phone is legendary,' someone said to me with a laugh just the other day.

Not having a smartphone, taking magic mushrooms, getting naked in the woods, and not washing — what cultural taboo was I going to break next? At this rate, I'd be Britain's most mocked man by the end of this book. I can picture *The Sun* headline now: 'Dirty hippy wants us to get naked, starve ourselves, and take drugs.'

I wasn't finished with the taboo-breaking, though. If doing without soap is one of our biggest cultural taboos, then I wonder where giving up toilet paper and talking about poo sits? I've been with my partner for 20 years, but I know there are some subjects she won't share with me. Talking about poo is one of the major ones; her mum was the same and her sister is, too. On the polar opposite side are my family: my mum seems to delight in telling me what foods do to her insides, and my dad could fart for England.

Considering it's something that can happen up to three times a day, I do think it's time we started a healthier conversation about it. So, let's start now: I want you to stop reading this book at the end of this paragraph and bookmark the page, returning only after you have had a poo. Of course, you might be sitting on the loo right now, 'dropping the kids off at the pool' — in that case, read on.

Excuse me for being personal, but how did that feel? As we've discussed, it's a difficult subject for many to approach — it's why we make up phrases like 'dropping the kids off at the pool', instead of just coming right out and saying 'having a poo'. Please don't be shy; it's just you and the page. You can share the details; pages don't talk. Although, if you are actually going to talk to the page and you are in a public place, you might want to check just outside the bathroom door in case someone is listening.

Okay, deep breath, and tell me: does it feel like there is a little bit left up there? Do you think you strained a little too hard? Was there even perhaps a bit of blood? Are these usual feelings when you go to the bathroom?

If you answered yes to one or more of the above questions, I might be able to help. The first of our problems begins with the toilet itself, especially if you sit on a Western-style toilet or even an East Asian bidet/toilet combo, complete with soothing music and bum drier. You see, toilets are quite a new invention; indeed, for most of humanity's existence, we didn't use them at all. We just squatted. For millions of years, that was the best way to poo.

In fact, there is some consensus forming that it still might be the best way to poo. Anything other than the squat position is detrimental, and Western toilets work against the natural functioning of our body. Your toilet might actually be bad for you.

For anyone who has heard of Giulia Enders, this information won't come as a shock. In her bestseller *Gut*, she cites the Dov Sikirov study of 28 test subjects.[32] Each participant was asked to poo in three different positions: firstly, sitting on a Western toilet, then half squatting on a very low toilet, and finally squatting over a hole. He then got them to record the time it took from — well, let's call it *blast off* — to landing. In the squatting positions, targets were landed in 50 seconds, and for those who were seated the length of time increased almost threefold to 130 seconds.

To understand why the height and shape of your toilet might affect your poo, imagine for a second the very end point of your Friday-night dinner, when it travels down through your colon, out of your rectum, and into the toilet. Think of the last bit, the out-of-the-rectum bit, as a trap door that must be opened and shut — the trap door is called the sphincter, and you have two of them, an inner and an outer one. When you sit normally, this trap door only opens a bit. When you squat, the trap door can be fully opened. If the door isn't fully opened, then there is extra strain on the body. Even tiny amounts of stress over a lifetime can wreck havoc on your rectum.

These bits of stress manifest as haemorrhoids, digestive diseases, and constipation, and they are more prevalent in countries that favour the Western-style sit-down toilet — of course, the Western diet doesn't help.[33] Apologies for the more graphic description, but too much pressure on the end of the gut means we can quite literally squeeze until our tissue comes out of our bum.

Just for balance, the squat toilet has come in for some criticism, too. Squat toilets are not great for those with knee problems or obese people, and although healthy on the bum, there does appear to be some evidence to suggest that blood pressure increases as we squat, and this might lead to strokes in the toilet — not the most pleasant place to check out of life.[34] However, the research seems to centre on a single study. So, in reality, it remains unclear whether squatting makes medically vulnerable people even more likely to have a heart attack than they would be when using Western toilets.

Before you rip out your toilet and replace it with a squat toilet, might I suggest a simple workaround? Place a small footstool in front of the toilet, put your feet on to it, and lean forward. This mimics the squatting position almost perfectly, at least enough to keep your rectum happy.

I try to do this in my house and have done for the last few years; although my daughter insists that the footstool is hers, and so it's not always where it should be. This innocent battle of the footstool has allowed me to frequently analyse my own toilet habits. What I have found is that the footstool works surprisingly well; it decreases the time I spend on the loo by about 50 per cent, and I feel like I push much less. There is often less to clean, too. On top of that, I make fewer visits to the toilet when I use it; I guess because I don't need to return to do a half-poo.

Overall, a simple footstool could be seen as a productivity and health aid all in one.

If you've ever been out hiking, cycling or camping in the wild and found yourself miles from any facilities, you may have first-hand knowledge of what is commonly known as a *wilderpoo*.[35] You might then also have an understanding of the best plants to use in this situation. Mullein, mallow, lamb's ear or even the Australian plant known as bushman's friend all have rather soft leaves and can become invaluable in a wilderpoo situation.

But why do we have to wipe when other animals don't? This is partly due to the shape, position, and mechanics of our anus — unlike many mammals, we have to wash or wipe. A horse, for example, has an anus that protrudes outwards when it poos, neatly retracting afterwards, negating the need for a wipe. But before you dog owners start shouting about your own dogs and their amazing ability to wipe their bums, think again. It might look like your dog wipes her bum when she pulls it across grass, but she doesn't. My apologies for making that action seem much less cute, and for ruining all those YouTube clips, but she is actually relieving fluid build-up in the anal gland.[36] Nice.

It might not seem fair that we don't all have magic self-cleaning bums, being the self-proclaimed dominant species and all. However, we humans traded that in when we started to stand upright and walk.

At this juncture, I must point out that our modern diet doesn't help matters. Think about the times you've done a ghost poo.[37] Those magical poos that don't need any bum-wiping. They are rare, right? Perhaps they were not so for our ultra-fit, squatting, non-processed-food-eating ancestors. Compare the ghost poo to its antithesis in modern poos, the ones that happen after a heavy night out. A night that included some sort of dirty takeaway food and alcohol. It's a question of chalk and rather runny cheese. Most of us have a lifestyle somewhere between these two extremes. Therefore, the ghost poo is rather elusive and, more often than not, we are left with the need to wipe or wash our bums.

For the majority of people in the UK, along with the USA and Australia, that means using dry toilet paper. Toilet paper and paper itself are thought to date back to around the second century BCE,[38] and back then its Chinese inventors would frequently suffer from splinters. Try not to spend too long thinking about that. Eventually, it made its way to the UK, before being exported out to North America and Australia. Historically, there have been many other ways we've removed poo from our bums. Some archaeologists believe that the Romans favoured a xylospongium, a sponge on a stick. In public toilets, this was shared but kept 'hygienic' by dunking it in a water, vinegar or saline solution.[39] Diseases were, of course, rife.[40]

Another option shared by early Romans and ancient Greeks was the pessoi — essentially, these were just stones that were the right size for the job. Meanwhile, over in ancient China and Japan, the hygiene stick was favoured. It could come in varying sizes, from chopstick-sized to much larger. These are perhaps good examples that modern innovation is not always a bad thing. So, toilet paper is an improvement on sticks, stones, and disease-ridden communal sponges, but is it the most ideal? Our bum is the most pathogenically troublesome area of our body, and around 30 per cent of the world's population cleans it with dry paper. As China and India become wealthier, this percentage might increase, bringing with it a host of problems.

To illustrate the first problem, I suggest a little experiment. You'll need a (willing) bearded person, some toilet paper, a cup of water, a hot day, and some chocolate buttons. Place the chocolate buttons on the beard of your willing volunteer and stand them out in the sun, allowing the buttons to melt. Once melted, try to wipe off the chocolate with toilet paper. Note how long it takes you.

I'm going to assume that you have amazing powers of persuasion if you got someone to volunteer for that little experiment. I'm also going to assume that your amicable bearded friend is perhaps feeling less amicable about the little bits of toilet paper and chocolate still in their beard. My final assumption is that they are asking for some water to wash their beard properly. Think about it: this is what we do with our bums on a sometimes thrice-daily basis. Does that sound like an effective solution?

It's not as if toilet paper is great for our anal health, either. Usage can lead to UTIs, chronic irritation of the vulva, haemorrhoids, and anal fissures. On a personal note, I also find my bum can be irritated if I eat the wrong foods or (as is my weakness) drink too much beer. This causes small spots of blood when using toilet paper, especially if I use it more than three times a day.

So then, what might be the alternatives?

My most favoured is the bidet. Whenever I travel to mainland Europe, I'm always delighted by the fact that there is a bidet (I've only ever seen one in a British home once). It makes me feel cleaner than using toilet paper, and the added bonus of a bidet is that it means I can enjoy spicy food again — another thing not to think about for too long.

Like most British people growing up through the 1970s and 1980s, I'd never even heard of a bidet, let alone seen one. My first encounter with one was on my first trip out of the country, the exotic delights of a camping holiday in France at age 11. I noticed a bidet in the local pizza restaurant, ironically called Crêpe et Pis, and my dad told me it was for washing your feet. For a decade, I thought the French were quite extravagant foot-washers. It wasn't until I briefly worked for KLM, the Dutch airline, and made tons of European friends, that I found out the truth. Pre-internet days in a provincial town were indeed the Dark Ages!

For those who've never come across one, a bidet is a kind of toilet-shaped sink with a mixer tap. Once you've finished having a poo, you turn on the tap and let the jet of water do its job, sometimes helping it on its way with a hand. You wash your hands afterwards and then either drip- or pat-dry your bum with a tiny amount of paper. I've found it hard to totally drop the use of paper and use a damp piece at the end to finish the job.

Women can also use a bidet when on their monthly cycle — to avoid having to have a full shower or bath — however, it's not to be used daily for this as the vagina cleans itself.[41] Lastly, you can indeed wash your feet in it — making my dad, at least a little bit, right.

At present, there are no peer-reviewed papers to argue the case for the health benefits of a bidet. The truth is, a little bit of poo left over isn't really going to cause any great problems. However, an estimated 1–5 per cent of the US population have *pruritus ani*, which is Latin for itchy anus. It's a condition that can be treated by removing the offending article of irritation;[42] this can be either toilet paper or a little bit of leftover poo.

I'd love to rush out and plumb in a bidet; however, my bathroom is like many city bathrooms and simply doesn't have the space for a bidet. Even if it did, Emma isn't quite as on board with the whole bidet idea as I am, and so it would be hard to justify the cost and inconvenience of installing one. Luckily, we live in a world where if there is a market, there is a product, and so there are a few alternatives.

These include various bidet attachments that can fit on to the existing plumbing on your toilet. They vary in luxury, from a simple shower nozzle with a cold single jet, to a fully heat- and pressure-controllable jet — although it is not advisable to penetrate the anus with water. The simplest, and by far the cheapest, is the portable bidet. These can be bought, or you could consider making your own. It is essentially a plastic bottle with a tube coming out of it. You squeeze the bottle and out comes the water. The results are mostly very good: when using this, I feel cleaner, I feel fresher, and I use around 90–95 per cent less toilet paper. Coupled with the stool-squat method, I feel like I poo better.

Sadly, after about six months of use, I stopped using the portable bidet, too. Our bath sits just in front of the toilet, close enough to be arm's reach away. I'd frequently leave the portable bidet in that spot, reminding Emma that I was using it, and she became less and less on board with the idea when confronted by it every time she used the loo. I can't blame her fully; it became a bit of an effort filling up the bottle and washing it every time. I'm left fantasising about a future where I can afford a bigger bathroom, one with enough room to fit in a foot washer!

If I'd lived before the Industrial Revolution — in fact, before farming — my diet would have been very different. There was no specific diet, as I'm talking about all humans across the planet over a vast amount of time. But what is true is the fact that I'd have had smaller meals with barely any fat, no sugar, and no or very little caffeine or alcohol, and they would also have included many more probiotic foods than we currently eat. I simply wouldn't have needed quite as much toilet paper. I certainly wouldn't have needed a bidet, as I'd have found myself with more solid poo. It all seems to come back to the idea that more stuff always leads to the need for more stuff.

What has been great for my wallet is that the amount of money I spend on cleaning myself has been stripped right back to the *bare* essentials. If I did have a bidet, too, and did without toilet paper, my bathroom bill would consist of the price of a bar of soap around twice a year. We fill our lives full of things that we don't need. Our nutrient-poor diet means many of us will buy supplements, too, and the pressures our society puts us under means we have to consume more medication. You might not take to all the things I mention in this chapter. But I would consider how much of your time and money is spent on grooming. If you are in the fortunate position to choose the number of hours you work, then think about how many of those hours are spent supporting your grooming habits. How many hours a week could you regain by reducing the time and money you spend on grooming?

What would you do with that extra time? Take up a hobby, maybe join an art class? Or perhaps try to concentrate on living longer.

When I was 39, I did exactly that. I was part of a group made up of around one in four adults who don't meet the recommended levels of physical activity. In fact, I was at the peak of my unfitness. I'd momentarily stumbled away from writing about plants into writing about beer, and it was starting to take its toll.

My other lifestyle choices didn't help much, either; I worked from a desk wedged into the corner of a box room, walked very little, and my bike sat gathering dust in the shed. I preferred instead to get taxis or the bus. I was drinking again, most nights; I ate a fried breakfast every morning, snacked on a chocolate bar or two every day, took sugar in my tea, and would eat out at every given opportunity.

I was in the obese category for the first time in my life. It showed, too: my trousers were popping buttons all the time and, although I'd ditched smoking a few years previously, I was still getting breathless walking upstairs.

That wasn't the worst of it. I had little energy for my family, including my new son, and I didn't have the energy to get to know anyone in the new area I'd moved to. I'm sure none of it helped my moods; dark, depressed days were frequent, and my ability to cope with stress dwindled. Dancing, cycling, and walking upstairs started to feel like an effort; I might have been 39, but my body was starting to feel like it was older — a lot older.

I consciously tried to make a difference to my size and fitness levels on many occasions; but this consisted mainly of buying fitness DVDs from charity shops and trying out a new wonder fitness regime in short bouts of two weeks, interspersed by trips to the pub, fried breakfasts, and cake. Needless to say, it wasn't enough, and for a while I kidded myself that I was living the 'good life'. The life of someone with money in the bank.

When I look up at my shelf of neglected fitness DVDs, I wonder why there are so many different diets and exercise regimes out there. If our natural way of being was to stay fit, there would be little need for them.

Sometimes I look at the local squirrels in the park and wonder if they ever worry about their weight. Every year, I notice lean and muscular-looking squirrels slowly getting really fat on acorns, and then these once agile creatures seem to struggle to get away from the local dogs. But far from being lazy, they put a lot of work into getting their acorns, morning, noon, and night, and in the autumn they can be seen gathering nuts or defending their territory. By the time my mind heads towards making acorn flour, they've scooped them all up, and they are proudly showing off their rather large bums — growing fat enough to stay alive through the winter.

I think about this sometimes as I travel, noticing that we'd prefer to act like supermarket groceries at the checkout when we visit airports, all of us lining up on that strange conveyor belt instead of walking. TV at the end of the day feels better than jogging, supermarket car parks are full and the footpaths are not, the stairwells in office blocks remain empty while the lifts are full, and if someone offers you a ride in their car, you are likely to say, 'Yes please.' Are we just naturally lazy?

Daniel Lieberman argues that this might be the case. In his book *Exercised*,[43] he argues that 'the instinct to avoid nonessential physical activity has been a pragmatic adaptation for millions of generations ... humans might have evolved to be especially averse to exercise' — suggesting that our ape-like cousins are even more inactive than we are. Silverback gorillas, for example, might have the odd fight, but they spend most of their time sitting on their sizeable bums, picking and eating leaves.

If I was going to lose weight, it had to be easier. The solution was around the corner. A shrinkage in income meant that I ditched the taxis and, as I live on part of a hill that is home to the steepest street in the UK, I really started to burn up the calories. I also now had two children and no car, which meant I walked with my son and pushed my daughter in her buggy with heavy shopping up and down that hill about four times a week. I couldn't afford to run a car, and Emma can't drive, so I'd also walk the 2.6-mile route to a greengrocer once a week, along with a few trips to the park and back, each time walking back up the steep hill with a buggy in tow. Lastly, I added a daily three-mile return trip to an office that I rented, via my children's school. It all added up — I estimate I walked about 30 extra miles (48 kilometres) each week — and I lost weight and got a little fitter.

Interestingly, I was naturally drawn to walk back the greenest way possible, either through the local park or up through a 44-acre Victorian cemetery, home to a small ash forest. When I walk that way, despite the hills being 1:4 in places, I rarely feel like I'm exercising. Turns out I might have stumbled across a way to make exercising feel less strenuous. In a study published in the *International Journal of Environmental Research and Public Research* in 2021,[44] 18 males were recruited and asked to do a sequence of wall squat exercises. A video of walking in a forest was played to some and a blank to others as a control. Their rate of perceived exertion was measured, along with their heart rate and other factors. The nature video not only lowered perceived exertion, but it also lowered their heart rate — What the study concluded is that being in nature increases the enjoyment of exercise.

Given that this was such a small study, I decided that I needed to put it to my own, rather crude, test. I picked up my dumbbells and found a three-minute dumbbell workout. I'd quickly flicked through about 50 workout videos to note that all of them had the trainer situated in a stark black or white minimalist gym, house or apartment. Other than a small vase of white flowers in one, none had people working out in any space that looked natural. In fact, none had anything that looked like a real home.

I never quite feel comfortable in houses that seem too perfect and sparse in furniture. I wondered if this was why, just ten seconds in, I felt a bit of strain. My eyes didn't leave the workout countdown, and my body seemed to ache with each move. I didn't feel like repeating it.

I rested for a day then did the same again. This time, I had a second screen playing a walk through a forest. I immediately felt a little more relaxed as I passed through a forest of larch trees, listening to birdsong, the gentle trudge of the cameraman's footsteps, and the trickle of the occasional stream. The noises and seeing the colour green both relaxed me, and I didn't look at the workout countdown at all. On reflection, I also think there was something else going on, enough distraction that I was not fully aware of my movements. It wasn't until two minutes in that I felt any kind of strain. After the workout, I felt jubilant, happy, and more energized. What was most surprising was that I felt like doing it again.

Had I lived in 1841, things might have been a bit different. I wouldn't have had to watch workout videos to get fit. My great-great-grandparents would have led a life that was similar to that of my 17-year-old active self. Back in the best decade, the 1990s, for a little over a year, throughout summer sun and cold wintery showers, I'd cycle five miles (eight kilometres) there and back to a clothes warehouse on the edge of town. Once there, apart from the 30-minute lunch break, I was on my feet for a whole eight-hour shift.

My 17-year-old self was lean, fit, but not overly muscular. My job then wouldn't have been too dissimilar to my ancestors' as, according to the 1841 census, a mere 0.1 per cent of the UK population had clerical jobs — that was approximately 18,500 people, which is less than the number of people currently working in video game development in the UK. The 1841 workers were a hardy bunch who didn't have labour-saving devices, either; carpets would have to be beaten, clothes scrubbed, tin baths carried and filled by hand and, perhaps worst of all, dishes washed without the aid of a dishwasher.

Even childcare was harder: on average, women had 4.85 children compared to 1.75 in 2020, and without disposable nappies, lightweight pushchairs, cars, and a more equal share of childcare between males and females, this meant a woman's lot was heavy lifting and carrying children over a longer period of her life.

Each labour-saving device we invent takes away a little more activity from our lives. I've noticed the change even in my lifetime: we can swipe a screen instead of walking a few metres to our central heating thermostat, and we message each other electronically instead of walking to a postbox. The internet has changed how we buy things, too; my home town of Northampton now has robots delivering local shopping, robbing us of even more exercise.

Compare this to how my generation bought things back in the 1990s. I'd walk about 0.8 miles (1.1 kilometres) to a video shop to rent a movie, and I'd travel about five miles (eight kilometres) on foot or cycle into town and back to get new clothes. If I wanted something really fancy, I might walk the extra mile to the train station and head across to Milton Keynes, the nearest city. I'd walk back from town on a night out at least five times a week, and I'd dance for at least an hour once there. To sound even more like an old man reminiscing about how hard life was, I can even remember buying computer games from a shop instead of downloading them. Watching TV before remote controls — something that appals my son. With phones in every pocket to watch TV on, even that tiny bit of exercise has been lost.

I'm not totally bemoaning the modern world, but current statistics suggest that with each extra inconvenience eliminated, we are getting less and less fit. Maybe packaging on every labour-saving device needs to come with a health warning: 'This product will reduce your exercise level by 30 kilocalories a day and reduce your life span; please replace with a five-minute jog once a week.'

Yet, as with much of the research into fitness, we only seem to look at it in reaction to poor health; we don't see fitness as the default setting it should be. So, aside from ensuring that mind and soul are in working order, what does being fit actually mean to a 21st-century human being?

Some fitness regimes, such as Paleo Fitness, Caveman Training and Crossfit Caveman, try to look further back in time, to mimic our ancestors. Often we might hear that 'our ancestors would run after prey until it fell down dead',[45] but did they? Let's think about it logically. Imagine we are in a merry band of Palaeolithic people. One of our crew, Derek, is really good at running; in fact, he is so good that it's his thing — he is known as that guy who runs after deer. Why would anyone else want to do it? Perhaps Derek and his mate Phil will each run after a deer and see who is best; perhaps they take it in turns. But does the whole group of 150 people run after deer? No. Some might be better at digging for roots, some at fishing, some at swimming or climbing for honey.

And that is exactly what played out when two of my old friends, Dan and Naomi, took part in the reality TV show I mentioned earlier, *Surviving the Stone Age*, where a group of specialists in ancient techniques survived for a month in the Bulgarian wilderness using only primitive technologies.

I asked Naomi about my Derek theory. It amused her, and she agreed, explaining that one of the group's survivalists and Stone Age experts, Matt Graham, could '... run barefoot up and down mountains. He could do it silently and not scare the animals or destroy any trails. He was the number one scout and would go ahead and we'd follow once he'd found a trail.' She went on to say, 'He loved it, and you couldn't really stop him. We all had our skill and personalities and we all found our niches.' Dan (her partner) would go off in the morning to hunt: he needed the calories and so off he went, forced out of bed by his stomach. She didn't like red meat and would not be as hungry in the morning, and so she stayed at the camp. Even within their small group, there wasn't a one-size-fits-all fitness regime, and it appeared that personal needs and preferences played a small but significant part in how much an individual exercised.

This dynamic plays out across the world with the wonderful diversity that is humanity. Consider those who lived around 40,000 years ago in what is present-day Japan. Evidence has been found for trap-pit hunting.[46] I can just imagine being part of this community, nipping off with a few mates for a day's foraging, or perhaps diving down into the ocean to pick shellfish off the sea floor, returning home just before dusk to collect a boar that had been caught in a trap. The food would have been plentiful and relatively easy to harvest. Whenever I've lived off wild food, it has always been near the coast — it's so much easier. This island race would have had a nutrient-dense diet and wouldn't have needed to run for miles on end, nor would they have needed to be overly muscular — boars were not carried for miles, as the traps were often found just outside settlements.

We could also mention the most studied group of hunter-gatherers around today, the Hadza of Tanzania. A recent study published in the journal *Nature Human Behavior* tracked the movements of a little over 2,000 Hadza foragers.[47] The study found that the adult Hadza men walked on average 18,476 steps, and the adult women 10,888 — that's 8 miles (12.9 kilometres) and 4.7 miles (7.6 kilometres) respectively. The women spend their time digging up roots and looking for plants, and the men hunt and climb trees for honey. When you drill down into the data, you'll find that it doesn't paint the whole picture. One man travelled a marathon distance at just under 27 miles (44 kilometres), while another was quite sedentary, travelling a little over 1.2 miles (2 kilometres). The outliers for women showed that some walked 0 miles and some up to 20 miles (32 kilometres) a day. They are as diverse a group as any.

So, what is right for us? What can we learn from our cousins in different countries, our ancestors, and present-day hunter-gatherers? The truth is, these people were, and are, as diverse and individual as you and me. The reason why there are so many of us around now is that we learned to adapt, live, and thrive in the most diverse of climates and conditions.

What we need to each ask ourselves, then, is what function does fitness serve for each of us as individuals? Are we living our best lives, and could exercise, in whatever form it might take, benefit us? The answer is yes, of course exercise can benefit us, and in fact some doctors are starting to call exercise the miracle cure and a wonder drug.[48] What I needed, and what I think one in every four humans on this planet needs, is to find that daily movement that fits our own lives.

For me personally, I want three things out of my fitness levels. I want to be healthy, happy, and still around to see my grandchildren. By that point, I'll be around 77, which is older than my parents are right now. I also want to be strong — strong enough to be of help with my grandchildren, to carry shopping bags across long distances, and to get the chance to pretend I'm good at DIY.

There is no getting away from the fact that I have a sedentary job. However, I can expect to add even more years on to my life when I start to add a little movement. Hannah Aram from George Washington University looked at the optimal dose for exercising and longevity.[49] Pooling data collected from over one million men and women in the United States and Europe, she looked specifically at the number of minutes of vigorous leisure-time activity. What she found is that with just 150 minutes a week, or 21 minutes a day, you will see your mortality rate reduce by 50 per cent — and that was across all ages. The benefit increases the more exercise you do, levelling off at about 1,000 minutes a week, or 142 minutes a day; after that point, there is little or no extra benefit. If this seems like a lot to cram into a working week, fear not: it appears that cramming all your physical activity into a weekend will see similar benefits.[50]

What kind of exercise, I hear you ask. I personally find that if you can include it in your daily routine, that really helps. The second thing is that you have to enjoy it. For me, that means walking. I love walking and frequently hop on a bus and walk the surrounding countryside, or take walking holidays. Even if I get to go on holiday with friends, or work away from home, I'll spend the mornings walking by myself while they spend their time relaxing. Yes, I know that might sound strange to some people, but I like nothing more than strolling through the countryside by myself and can do it for hours on end without really feeling like I'm exercising.

But this love of walking means it doesn't feel like too much extra effort to take a slightly longer walk back after dropping the kids off at school. I can also take a route with the most greenery, as I mentioned, as this helps to increase my enjoyment and lower my perceived level of effort. As the school is at the bottom of my hill, it means any walk back involves a bit of a climb — good news for my heart, as this really can get it pumping.

But should I be running a little? Judging by the amount of Lycra and bouncing ponytails I see at pick-up time, running is the most popular exercise at our kids' school. Seeing that abundance of healthy-looking people always makes me feel like I should be doing more. But running has never been my thing. Every year I aim to try it, but I still haven't erased the horror of that run on a cold November afternoon at my middle school. I know I have a mental block, but should I be working on it?

Well, yes and no. Running is excellent cardio, but so is walking. I'm not saying you should stop if you love running — far from it. I do understand that beyond the obvious health benefits, the runner's high is real, and that it can be a great bonding thing to train with someone else. Instead, I will speed up my walk slightly, and, according to the catchily named AHA journal *Arteriosclerosis, Thrombosis, and Vascular Biology*,[51] the equivalent energy expenditures of moderate walking and vigorous running produce similar reductions in the risk of hypertension, hypercholesterolemia, diabetes, and possibly even chronic heart disease. Or, in plain English, if I speed-walk, especially uphill, it has similar benefits to running. Not only that, there can be up to a 70 per cent chance of injury when running compared to a 1–5 per cent chance while walking.[52] This is music to my ears: I can walk and still increase my chances of living for longer, and perhaps feel a little smug about it, too.

Walking has other benefits. With so many of us now working from home, I believe a simple routine that involves a walk will improve performance and wellbeing. Einstein, too, had a daily walking ritual, which was sacrosanct.[53] As did the great American naturalist, poet and philosopher Henry David Thoreau, who stated: 'Methinks that the moment my legs begin to move, my thoughts begin to flow.'[54] It appears that science agrees with these great minds, and your brain might actually work better when you add physical activity.[55] Rodents that are given free access to a running wheel show a remodelling of the brain that leads to improved memory,[56] prolonged cognitive longevity, and reduced risk of dementia.[57]

More good news (for me) is that, according to Dr Pedro

Saint-Maurice, the positive effects of exercise will still be felt even if hitherto sedentary 40–61-year-olds start to increase their exercise levels. He cites a level of about seven hours a week — that's an hour a day of fast walking. If I add a half-hour evening walk to my routine, this is more than achievable.

One thing I've noticed is that giving up or reducing the amount you drive or sit on a bus is possibly one of the healthiest things you can do. I've dusted off my bike and use that for anything over two miles (3.2 kilometres); otherwise, I walk. It's working, too: today I bought myself a smaller pair of jeans. I've gone down two sizes — I've not been that size for 20 years! It's taken about three months to lose four inches off my waist, and that is mostly from walking more. As I'm 174 centimetres (5 feet 8.5 inches) tall, this means my height-to-waist ratio (waist circumference ÷ height) is 0.47, which is now way below the 0.52 healthy limit for men; in fact, it's even below the 0.48 healthy limit for women. A study in *The Journal of Clinical Endocrinology and Metabolism* considers this number to be a better predictor in reducing the risk of diabetes, heart disease, and stroke for both men and women.[58] What's more, my blood pressure is now at an ideal level, too, without the need for medication.

I had to find something I enjoyed, or I would have stayed at an unhealthy weight, and I'm not alone. Marie Dacey et al looked at this issue back in 2008.[59] Taking a study of 645 adults, they concluded that intrinsic motivation and self-determined extrinsic motivation distinguish older adults' activity levels. Or, in other words, you have to like whatever you are doing to be motivated to do it.

NEW WILD YOUR BODY

It's easy to wean yourself off a detergent-based cleaning regime. Introduce soap for one day a week, then two days the next week, until you are using just soap. Then slowly transition away from using it on your body.

I choose to continue to use soap on my hands in order to reduce the spread of disease. I also continue to use it in areas that could smell.

Each hair type is different. Consider using just soap before switching to a water-only regime. Comb your scalp frequently to avoid the build-up of any residue, and use diluted apple cider vinegar if dandruff becomes a problem.

Bring a pile of books or a footstool into your bathroom and leave it next to the loo. Footstools can often be picked up second-hand.

When it comes to exercise, I'm not you, and I can't tell you what you should be doing. But if you want to change something, to live a longer and healthier life, I'd suggest trying everything until you find something you enjoy, then stick to it.

It may be wise to give up sugar. This can be harder than you think. Prepare a week beforehand by looking at the all the triggers, such as every time you are near certain shops, if you saw a biscuit tin open, or if you have a coffee. This will prepare you for when you do quit, then take long deep breaths instead until the craving has passed. Don't beat yourself up if you slip up and succumb to a craving.

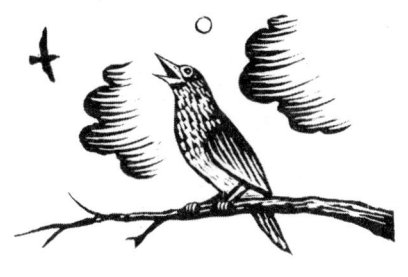

CHAPTER FIVE

Music

'But the drumming and the dreaming still goes on, the wind still whispers from the spirit land'

C.E.S. WOOD, 1880

Once I decreased how much time, and money, I spent in the bathroom, I started to think about other aspects of modern city living that weren't benefiting me.

I had a glimpse of a less modern world when I visited rural Romania not long after the Berlin Wall fell and took the European communist experiment with it. It was a time of great economic hardship. For a young visitor, not caught up in the trials and tribulations of trying to make a living in a harsh economic climate, and perhaps being less sensitive to what was going on around me, there was a sense of serenity. I can remember sitting on a mountain, a town nestled in the valley below me. I soon realised that the only noises I could hear were animals: goats, horses, and the odd dog or two. They were accompanied by birds of prey overhead and, one night, the howl of a wolf. We were told that bears might live in these woods — far from being scared, it felt natural, normal. Similar, perhaps, to the soundscape here in the UK before the Industrial Revolution. Although I wasn't about to explore the woods.

I think about that time when the magnitude of man-made noises in this city makes me feel hemmed in. I can't turn back time, nor can I convince everyone to jump on a bike, walk or simply slow down their lives and enjoy their surroundings without rushing off. Instead, I sometimes close the window and play a recording of birdsong to put me in a different headspace. The sound reminds me of my childhood home, the sanctity of our long and wooded garden, which was often alive with birdsong and the noise of squirrels.

Emerging evidence from the UK, Norway, and the Netherlands suggests that drowning out the noise of the road with more natural sounds can help us stay trim.[1] Long-term exposure to traffic noise has been linked with a larger girth due to an increased level of stress hormones.[2] More alarmingly, exposure to loud noises can lead to resistant hypertension — high blood pressure that is resistant to medication.[3] It's not good news for anyone suffering from heart trouble, either,[4] as evidence is emerging to suggest that long-term exposure to loud noise may lead to an increase in cardiac fibrosis, a condition that creates too much collagen around the heart, restricting it in doing its job. In other words, traffic is not just damaging our lungs through air pollution, it is damaging our hearts through noise pollution, and that is to say nothing about how much it is damaging our environment or how dangerous it is.

Just listening to birdsong can help, though. Sometimes I do this in the form of a YouTube video when I can't escape my desk. But I wonder: is it enough? Dr Eleanor Ratcliffe, an environmental psychologist from the University of Surrey, can help to answer that.[5] She questioned 174 British people after playing them the song of 50 different birds. She found a positive response to many of the songbirds from those participants who enjoyed spending time outdoors. They reported finding the noises restorative, that they improved their mood and cognitive performance. It would appear, then, that in listening to birdsong, I'm giving my brain a bit of a mental massage.

The birdsong relaxes me, puts me in a calmer state of mind. I look out of the window at the walnut tree in our back garden. The tree is still young for a walnut tree; I can remember around 11 years ago, when we first moved in, seeing the squirrel that planted it hopping along the back fence with a mischievous lilt to his movements. That squirrel gave us a beautiful shaded place to eat in the summer and the best climbing tree around for our and the neighbourhood kids. It almost feels like a bonus, too, that we get food from this tree. Having lived in cities for most of my adult life, a garden big enough to have any tree feels like a blessing, and this year I've started emulating the squirrel, distributing the nuts to any gardener who promises to grow the tree's offspring. If I am to continue to restrict this tree's natural growth when she offers so much in return, it seems only fair.

I think of the future as I pass on these small,

golf-ball-sized nuts, of how they brim with the potential to start a succession of trees which could feed the generations that follow me. I wonder if that squirrel knew exactly what he was doing as he buried the nut. I wonder if the idea that nut-burying animals simply forget where they buried their nuts is an arrogance on our part, if actually they plan for their future, intentionally planting a few nuts so that their offspring can eat. I've watched the local squirrels as they stand on top of fence posts in the local cemetery; the ones that don't appear to notice me have a faraway look, and if I didn't know any better, I'd say it looks like they are daydreaming. But they are far more in tune with their surroundings than we are. There is an intelligence we can't fathom within that small rodent head and body.

A wistful part of me imagines that the drumming noise the squirrels make when running along the fence is intentional, that they are creating a deliberate drumbeat. After all, percussive sound is powerful and persuasive; I know that from my early experiences of acid house.

Considering percussive sound's power leads me in an interesting direction. It's the first sound that any of us hear and feel, as it's the sound of our mother's heartbeat. We might hear plenty of sounds outside the womb, but they are muffled, like hearing something from another room. Our mum's heartbeat, however, is constant, strong — it sounds like an underwater kick drum.[6] This beat is working to help form a powerful bond. At about a month after fertilization,[7] a foetus' heart has formed enough that it can start pumping blood. From this point onwards, rhythmical breathing can bring both heartbeats into synchronisation.[8] This calms both the mother and baby, but also, this ability to synchronise our hearts might help us to socialise in later life. It's found that those who suffer from social anxiety have an inability to synchronise heartbeats with those around them.[9] Could percussive sound help?

Forming a bond with our children is undeniably important in the survival of species. But percussive sound can also help to form a bond with a place. I remember taking a six-hour train journey up to Edinburgh, my first visit to Scotland. It was August, at the tail end of the world-famous festival, and when I left the station, I heard the sound of drums and bagpipes filling the air. The back of my neck tingled, my heart pounded to the beat; the atmosphere was electric. A bond was formed: Edinburgh now had a special place in my heart — in fact, for a short while after, we started looking for houses up there and almost moved.

What I was feeling wasn't something only felt by tourists who have had a great holiday; it was something that humans have felt for thousands of years, maybe since before we had language to describe it.[10] At the moment, we can only speculate that other hominids, such as Neanderthals,[11] may have been drummers. That speculation is fuelled when we look at our chimpanzee cousins,[12] who use a form of drumming, beating out rhythms on the roots of trees — the resulting sound sends reverberations across forests over distances of up to 0.6 miles (1 kilometre). Each chimp will have their own signature drumming pattern — a beat that is all their own — informing other chimps where they are and what they are doing. What I find fascinating is just how excited this practice makes them — hooting and screeching as they drum out a few beats. It feels like the excited email or text you might send a friend after you've had a particularly good night out with them. A form of social bonding.

Granted, the beats are short; you couldn't call them a language. Yet, drumming can convey much longer and more complex messages. The Bora people of Peru and Colombia use huge drums called manguaré to mimic the entirety of their language, the number of beats matching the number of syllables.[13] The beats act like short text messages; each message consists of about 60 drumbeats, which then translate into a 15-word sentence.

This isn't the only language that can be tapped out in a rhythm. Morse code is in essence a drumbeat language. Once skilled, you can tap out around 12 words per minute. It was extensively used during World War II to send messages across radio waves, and it's still taught by the SAS.[14]

Percussive sound, then, might be useful for bonding and communication, too; perhaps this is why it is hard-wired into our DNA. Indeed, as soon as a foetus' inner ear has fully developed and hearing starts, at 26 weeks, we start to react to drums and drumming. The heartbeats of babies can change when they hear music inside the womb.[15]

This continues to happen once a child has been born, and many babies will move once they start to hear a beat.[16] It might not always be what we'd consider dancing — that ability comes later, and some of us never quite get it — but most children over the age of two and a half will move in time with a beat,[17] and adjust their movement accordingly to match the rhythm of the drummer.[18]

One of my dearest and oldest friends, Sarah Larkham, an author, musician, artist, and charity worker from Bristol, co-runs a charity founded by her husband, Elliot Hall, called Mind Your Music. I spent the morning with her, quizzing her about a drumming session she coordinates and facilitates for people with a variety of mental health problems.

> We have socially anxious people, mainly. Ours is maybe the one social contact they have. Some of them are really anxious and some of them are hyper. And we teach specific rhythms; it's not like we start drumming and they join in, as that would be chaotic and quite challenging to people who don't have any confidence in themselves. So we give really specific patterns. When they all get that, we split the group and then play two together. You have to concentrate so much on that sound you are holding that you don't have any room in your mind for intrusive thoughts. That's how it works.
>
> That's how shamanic drumming is, too. Its repetitive rhythm becomes the only thing — the only thing you're aware of ... and even when I'm teaching the drums — this happened last week — I close my eyes and get into the rhythm so much that I forget I'm supposed to be responsible for people, because it's carried me away so much. So by the time we've done 45 minutes of drums, maybe an hour, we can then start teaching songs, singing, and instruments ... and it means people aren't afraid anymore to sing in front of others.

I wondered how this might have worked when I was younger, if instead of starting off the school day with a register, an act that highlights individuality, then setting a bunch of academic tasks — tasks that rank us in order of how well we perform, further adding to a feeling of division — we instead had started with something that unified us, calmed us. That instead of making us stand up on our own to read something out, we had joined in together. I, of course, felt awkward; I wondered if most of the kids did. However, it would have taken a Herculean effort on behalf of the school and teachers even to suggest music lessons every day. It was a subject that was never taken seriously at my school; we all considered it a doss lesson.[19] None of us really saw how it related to our own lives. But it did unite and uplift us — could it be that music was one of the more important lessons, after all?

Sarah then told me how it affects her and the group after a session:

> We're often really busy, and to get to a venue we have to drive through horrific traffic, and so we tend to arrive quite fraught. We then have to set everything up, and it does feel like work. By the time the group has left, we've been on a journey together, and it doesn't feel like work anymore. It's something we've shared and we can't wait to do it again. Everyone's on a bit of a high, and it definitely feels like an achievement. It's a social high, I suppose; it feels deeper than that, though ... the bond that it's created is what's kept our organisation going for 20 years.

Then she said something even more remarkable that will stay with me: 'I've seen people who are mentally comatose have conversations after drumming.'

I may not be mentally comatose, but since moving out of a shared office environment, and having less social time due to looking after Khloe, I've grown increasingly aware that my social skills are becoming rusty. Don't get me wrong; I'm the king of chitchat — I sometimes examine shop workers as they serve me in order to find something I can strike up a conversation about, telling them they have interesting earrings or asking people with blue hair if that is their natural colour. I stop people in the street and chat about their dog, the dark cloud above us, or how great their shoes are. If I'm rehearsed, I can give talks to hundreds. However, put me in a room with more than two people — or fewer than 500 — when I've been writing a lot and socialising less, and I suffer. The thought of being part of a group dynamic, but not having to talk to them all, really appealed.

The appeal was so strong that it led me to a platform at a tiny Wiltshire railway station. I stood there clutching a map, trying to work out if I really did need to walk up that very steep hill in front of me. I asked the one other person who had got off at the same station. She seemed pleased to chat; I assumed that conversation was a rarity at this request-only stop. She directed me to the village that sat high above us, and I started my ascent to a village hall in the middle of nowhere — the closest drumming circle to my home that I could find.

As I walked, I started to feel a little nervous. I was about to walk into a room full of strangers who already had established relationships with each other, to play an instrument that I had no idea how to play. I did my best to turn that nervousness into excitement; the body doesn't know the difference, after all. Both anxiety and excitement are aroused emotions and, however you frame it, the body displays the same levels of feeling. Writing in *The Atlantic*, Olga Khazan cites various studies claiming that reframing nervous feelings as excitement will improve performance.[20] I used to get wound up with nerves before talking in public. But since reframing the experience as an exciting one that I'm pleased to say, things have turned around. However, in this case, nerves were winning, and so I sat, ate a quick sandwich, and contemplated why I might be working this situation up in my mind.

It had been a very tough year. I was still writing two books at once and looking after Khloe, though thankfully her health had been improving day by day, and I had been taking care of my mental health, too, with my experiments.

I thought about a local parent I'd seen caring for a child with highly demanding additional needs. Like many of the unpaid care workers around the country, she looked like she needed a break. But admitting you need time off comes with guilt. It's such a knotty thing, caring, in our society that is structured around getting us working and not helping us to help each other.

Khloe was still wobbly at times, but her condition continued to improve. A day or two before, she had started to clap out a rhythm, chanting 'cha cha cha' as she did so. She urged us to join in, and of course we obliged, dancing together on the tiny strip of space on the upstairs landing, which has barely enough room to turn — but it was so much fun. I had to hide my tears as we danced, to save them from being misinterpreted as sorrow. Those were the first steps I'd seen Khloe take in six months.

We are a close family and try to be a caring one; we all work at keeping it so. The clapping helped to reinforce our bonds, as mimicry works as a social glue.[21] As I walked up that hill, I pondered that moment and how it had brought us together, how it had made caring easier for all of us. I suspected the drum circle might do the same; it was certainly what Sarah thought, too. I wondered if the drumming would help to form bonds, just like the hand-clapping had. The questioning side of my brain then wondered if I might find the whole experience underwhelming, if I was putting too much emphasis on the 'magic' of the drum, if I was expecting too much.

After an hour walking uphill, I arrived at a fairly large village hall. Architecturally, it looked like it was from the 1940s, wooden and perfunctory, but inside it was freshly painted and welcoming. Three people sat there, each with a massive drum in front of them and big friendly smiles on their faces. The one woman had to be Michelle, I thought, the main organiser who'd agreed to lend me a drum for the evening.

'Are you Michelle?' I asked.

'Yes,' she said.

I motioned to the untouched drum next to her. No response. I felt uneasy — had she changed her mind? Was I meant to bring a drum? My heart rate increased, my hands became clammy and my voice shaky. This was going to be awkward: a whole evening in a drum circle without a drum. Then another woman came in and everyone greeted her as Michelle. The first woman turned out to be called Jan. Jan obviously hadn't heard me properly — perhaps due to a lifetime of drumming. Eventually, the real Michelle did give me a huge djembe drum, telling me with a smile that the word 'djembe' derives from the saying 'anke djé, anke bé', which means 'everyone gather together in peace'.[22] I liked that. This was a better start.

The djembe is a West African goblet drum designed

to be played with your hands. They vary in size, but I estimated that all the djembes in that room were at least 60 centimetres (nearly 2 feet) tall with a 30–40-centimetre (12–16-inch) diameter. Mine was heavy, and I was shown how to strap myself in, literally tying myself to this drum. It felt somehow comforting and reminded me of how, when they were tiny, I used to strap my children to me in their carriers whenever we left the house. It felt like I was bonding with my drum.

Without warning or explanation, the group started to hammer out a rhythm. I joined in and, much to my own astonishment, I could keep up. It really should have felt like a baptism of fire — I'd never had drumming lessons, after all — but it wasn't. Here I was, keeping time with people who'd drummed all their lives. I kept to the beat throughout that first tune, a full five minutes of drumming, and felt joyous. I mean, I was still a little uptight and nervous about missing a beat, but the fact remains that I didn't.

I felt like I was running in a race. Yet, it was more than that, much more: it felt like I was truly alive, free of my general anxiety and everyday worries. I'd never even dreamed it would be like this. The setting didn't matter; it drifted away. I had expected to feel nervous and self-conscious but, while I was drumming, that went away. On more than one occasion, I got so lost in the beat that I carried on when the others stopped, and I didn't care!

I wasn't a perfect drummer, and occasionally I dropped beats and fell out of rhythm with the group. I especially found it difficult to get into First Nation rhythmic patterns, and during the more complex rhythms at the end. I also remained a little self-conscious at times, but I could see this changing as I got to know the group. However, for a good three-quarters of the time, I was mostly lost in the frenzy of it all. We played a mix of beats, mostly West African in origin, and some with rhythmic singing, too. At one point, Michelle pulled back, turning the beat into something slower — intimate, even. Smiles were shared around the room; it was as if we were speaking a different language — a wordless, ancient language.

After we finished, there was some chat among the group. It was casual, and I felt closer to the people in that room. I noticed that I'd become fully relaxed in the company of everyone. Sarah was right: it felt as if we'd been on a journey together. I could really see how this would help teams of people struggling to find common ground; the act of drumming together became the common ground, breaking all class, economic, sexual orientation, and racial barriers.

I had no idea of the background of anyone in the group. If I was to stereotype from their appearances, I was sitting with a retired general, a graphic designer, an actuary, a botanist, and a salesman, but really I had no idea, and it just didn't matter. There was a real atmosphere of inclusion, giving, and acceptance — powerful stuff! The talk between them all was of drumming; they were organising musical meet-ups at each other's houses, and I was made to feel welcome should I wish to join them. They were warm and gentle with each other — we had gathered together in peace.

Jan drove me back to the station and, as she did so, she told me about her life — how she'd worked in festivals and lives on a boat — but this felt like icing. It was nice to hear, but I felt I'd met her on a different level. I thought back to one glorious night when I had danced until dawn in a

London club. I was in the centre of a room and, as I danced, I looked up to see faces smiling at me. As far as I could see across the dance floor, everyone was smiling. I spun around to find the whole room was facing my way, and we all exchanged the most heartfelt smiles. I might have been too shy to approach any of those people in daily life back then — they were cool Londoners, after all, and I was a provincial boy; I felt in awe. Yet, on the dance floor, some connection was made. I could be the centre of attention, and it just felt like we were all connecting. It was natural. I'd always thought it was down to the drugs, but maybe the drums had their influence, too?

Neither my experience nor Sarah's is particularly unusual when it comes to drumming and drum circles. The feeling of connectedness is a common theme and one that is used as a powerful therapeutic tool in the mental health practitioner's toolkit, not just to help those who are suffering, but also to aid cohesion between them and their carers. Indeed, when 39 service users, carers, and psychologists from the same mental health setting started to drum together,[23] the results were certainly very favourable. Participants reported not only increased feelings of wellbeing, but also an increased sense of control over their lives, a sense of accomplishment, increased self-acceptance, and a more positive view of the world. They also found that 'changes in well-being through music can go beyond the private individual level, and are sufficiently empowering to build strong connectedness and promote openness, agency, and social engagement'.

This last point I find very pertinent. I worked in a mental health setting 20 years ago as a health care assistant on a locked ward. I met some truly remarkable people, both staff and service users. However, as with every workplace, there were alliances and sometimes quite bitter divisions. Years of underfunding did nothing to ameliorate this issue, leading to occasions of bed-blocking, violent people thrown in with the clinically depressed and vulnerable, and dangerous levels of understaffing.[24] In this atmosphere, it was hard to see how a culture of distrust *wouldn't* arise.

I wonder how different the situation would have been if we'd drummed together? I know it sounds rather naive, because it wouldn't have undone the underfunding or changed the admissions procedure. However, anything that builds a sense of openness and support would have been preferable to the culture I eventually felt forced to leave.

The very real sense of openness and support that drum circles offer opens the door to new possibilities with groups. In one study, drug addicts looking for a release from their suffering turned to drumming.[25] When counselling fails, a sense of community can help to replace feelings of isolation, alienation, and self-centredness. It also gives people a high, and offers social support in a secular setting.

But group bonding isn't the only reason I am interested in drumming. At one point during Michelle's drum circle, between beats, someone held up a beater and wanted to use it. 'No, no — that's something quite different,' said Michelle with a dream in her eyes. 'That's a beater for a shamanic drum.' I liked the sound of that, the *shamanic drum*, and I promised myself it would be the next thing I tried.

Our routes to things can come from the strangest of sources. As a teenager, I got into a group called The Shamen, a band remembered more for their pop songs like

'Ebeneezer Goode' and 'Move Any Mountain' than anything else. Yet, they introduced me to a lot of shamanistic concepts, including psychedelic experimentation and the shamanic use of a drum. Their song 'Boss Drum' spoke of connections with the goddess, altered consciousness, and eternal rhythms for future generations. Maybe the future generation was now?

I kept my eyes open for a drum. Then, rather cheaply, I picked up a bodhrán' from a charity shop and, rather expensively, a beater from a shop in Glastonbury. I batted out a very simple beat of one note, hammered out on the drum. It was soothing, but not life-changing. Then I found a video of a drum being beaten, accompanied by the sound of a bullroarer.[26]

The bullroarer is a simple instrument consisting of a small (20–30 centimetre) carved piece of wood. It's shaped like a surfboard but with a point at both ends, and you tie it to a piece of cord. It is 'played' by spinning it in circles through the air, and the air resistance makes a kind of other-worldly humming sound. Those old enough might remember one being used as a 'phone' in the 1986 Paul Hogan film *Crocodile Dundee*.[27]

I lay on my bed with my eyes shut, listening to the sounds. I naturally found myself focusing in on the sound of the drum and nothing else. Within moments, I could feel a twitch coming from my stomach, and soon my whole body was convulsing. It felt like the drum was being played from inside me. When my stomach stopped twitching, my legs took up the beat, as if they were being invisibly shaken by some external force. It was odd — very odd — but it wouldn't be the oddest thing that's happened to me recently.

If you look across antiquity, from First Nation and Aboriginal culture to ancient China and prehistoric Britain, you'll find drums at the heart of many ceremonies. Yes, they are bonding, and, yes, the sound of a drum can rouse emotional states. But in my experience, they can also lead to altered states of consciousness.

Shamanic drumming typically consists of repetitively beating a drum at around four to five beats a second.[28] This beat can be enough to induce 'a trance-like state', and 'in the extreme case, twitching of the body and a generalized convulsion are reported'.[29] It is thought that such behaviour results from a stimulation of the nervous system. These altered states of consciousness are similar to those we get when using psychedelic substances, when meditating, or when running long distances. These are known as *hypnodal states*, and a scale has been developed to measure them. In the Phenomenology of Consciousness Inventory,[30] drumming is measured as inducing an average level of trance, falling within the medium range of consciousness-altering experiences.[31]

I wanted to experience this more fully. I put the track on again and closed my eyes, visualising myself in a beautiful natural setting, finding a foxhole and climbing inside, as directed by Irish shaman Martin Duffy.[32] I am not sure it made a huge difference compared to just closing my eyes, but it was pleasant nonetheless.

I've now practised these drum trips a number of times, and each time differs. However, what is constant is a feeling that someone else is present, a feeling I also had during my experience with the mushrooms and during my utiseta.

As I have been discovering my New Wild Order, I have

found myself reframing my past. Perhaps my childhood was not as bad as I sometimes remember it. Yes, I was anxious, but that didn't define me. It wasn't all I was. I think that, at times, I've forgotten this and become locked in repeated thought patterns that recall only the bullying and loneliness, rather than the fun. The drums have helped me to remember the joy I felt, too. On one drum trip, I felt like I was on top of an Astroglide, a huge multi-sloped slide that you went down on a mat. I was filled with excitement, standing at the top, waiting my turn, mat in hand, and the sun was beaming down. I retained that feeling of excitement and joy long after the trip. I still feel happy and lighter recalling it as I type!

I did wonder if this was all in my head, a psychosomatic response. Then I discovered academic and prehistoric sound expert Paul Devereux. Devereux suggests that drumming can affect localised parts of the brain. One study suggested that as participants' drumming improved, so did their behaviour. Participants showed a significant reduction in hyperactivity and increased brain connectivity in the areas of the brain that help to inhibit impulses, evaluate choices, and regulate emotions.[33] Or, in other words, drumming helped these areas of the brain to function better. Perhaps areas of my brain that hadn't connected up since my childhood were again linking.

I wondered what else drumming might help with and found Laurel Hurst,[34] ethnomusicologist, registered nurse, and author of the 'Groove Therapy' TEDx Talk. She suggests that just two months of weekly drumming sessions helps the stress hormone cortisol to drop, along with increasing the anti-inflammatory cytokine IL-4; it also helps to increase serotonin and dopamine. In other words, drumming makes us happier and healthier. Science says so!

Paul supports the theory that sound might have played a bigger part in our day-to-day lives in ancient times than it does now. He suggests that sites like Stonehenge could be played like a giant glockenspiel — even the thought of being witness to that sound, while the winter sun rises after the longest night, makes the hairs on the back of my neck stand to attention.

Furthermore, he notes that ancient British burial sites are designed in such a way that a drummer can stand outside the chamber to allow a visceral effect of drumming on our bodies without hearing the drum. That drums are used in some First Nation ceremonies in the grieving process to 'bridge the link between life and death' only adds weight to this theory.

This morning, I walked Khloe into school. It feels good to write that. She still goes in a little later than the other children — a precautionary measure, really. It means that the roads are a little quieter and we are less likely to be interrupted with the tiny chats typical of the school run that tire her out. It also gives us a bit of time and space together. It's a highlight of my day. This morning, she was in a great mood and just started making noises — kind of singing, like the backing vocals in an a cappella arrangement.

One thing I've noticed as I have pieced together this New Wild Order is just how much of it is intuitive. How much of it we need to relearn from childhood. When I stopped using furniture for a while, I also went without shoes. My son and I walked to the shop barefooted, a distance of about one mile (1.6 kilometres) — something he does throughout the summer months (and would throughout the winter if we didn't make him wear shoes for fear of frostbite). He looked at me and said, 'Daddy, I think you are just learning to be me.'

He, too, has been making up little songs since he could talk. Most days, he'll sing something and, if I'm feeling relaxed and happy, and have the headspace, I do the same. So do Emma, Khloe, and my daughter. Anything can become a little song: shopping lists, requests for tea, or ballads sung with a conciliatory nature — *How can you forgive me for breaking your cup ... how can you forgive me when you cup lies there broke-n?**

I might not be much of a composer, or a singer, but music and song have always been important to me. Sometimes I dream whole tunes complete with visuals.

Music can literally make you weep. But weep with tears of what? Crying isn't a singular emotion. The last song I cried to was Saint Etienne's 'Hobart Paving'.[35] It gets me almost every time, or at least it did, especially when I felt a little broken, as I did a few years ago. This is backed up by the findings of a study published in the *Empirical Studies of the Arts* journal.[36] They suggest that people who feel sadness when they cry might score highly on the neurosis scale, while those who cry with awe are more likely to score highly as open individuals. I think I've stumbled on my own personal Saint Etienne neurosis scale. If I fall into bad habits and forget what I've learned, then I'll have to check in with that song!

I discovered Saint Etienne on BBC Radio 1. The radio

---

* Sung to the tune of Michael Bolton's classic 'How Can We Be Lovers'.

has always been an important piece of kit for me, and I now listen to a mix of UK, Australian, French, and US stations. Being able to tune into these stations would have blown my youthful mind. But even the static-filled pirate stations of my youth opened up the world up to me, feeling in some ways like rebellion. The radio was something I discovered, something that was just mine. I didn't have to share it as I did most of my toys — the joy of having a twin! It was something that took me out of the dreariness of Northampton in the 1980s, a place where suburbia could feel infinite.

The radio was a window to the new world of electronic music; where I first heard that sweeping synth at the start of Laura Branigan's 'Gloria', and the frantic genius of Gershon Kingsley's 'Popcorn', along with the ballads, rock music, and my beloved disco that drifted to my radio from the North Sea. These people were singing and playing for me. I have a warm feeling as I remember the C90 cassette tapes that housed these tracks, mixtapes I painstakingly created over weeks and months. If I happen to hear any of the songs from those tapes, I half expect to hear, in the background, the faint and ghostly broadcast from the French radio stations whose signals were being jammed. That music has embedded itself deep within me.

As a teenager and in my twenties, songs became anthems that I'd sing with friends and my brother: Bon Jovi, Iron Maiden, and Def Leppard all signalled a departure from childhood. I sang The Waterboys and N.W.A to mark the years of my most rebellious youth. These were the songs that bonded my crew and marked our territory. I had my first kiss to Bruce Willis's 'Under The Boardwalk'. As I grew, The Smiths, the Stone Roses, and Saint Etienne were chanted beside many a bar, and they are songs I can still sing to my friend Bez to make years of limited contact disappear. Break-ups had their own theme music, too; Jason Donovan's 'Too Many Broken Hearts' can still take me back to being 15 and the raw grief I felt when Alison Loveday dumped me to be with her ex again. One chorus of 'Gloria' and I'm back in the front room of my parents' house in 1982. I can smell the smells, feel the emotions; I know the colour of the curtains and settee, and all the other tiny details I'd forgotten come flooding back to me. My taste and choice in much might be unique, but the feelings these songs give me are not. Music and song persist across all cultures; in all likelihood, they have also existed across time. Why, then, has music always been so important to us?

There are a few theories out there, and what you have to remember about science is that, much like art, it reflects the time, culture, and personality of the person who created or theorised it. This book, for instance, reflects my personality. The subjects I've chosen, my worldview, are of someone born to Baby Boomer parents in a Midlands town. Of someone who was positively influenced by disco as a child, then rave culture as an adult, and someone who has never fitted into mainstream culture. I already know the people who'll appreciate this work and those who will reject it. Artists and scientists do not exist in a vacuum and, as such, any scientific theories are a reflection of that. This always needs to be considered when thinking about someone's theories or works.

I'm reminded of this when I think about Lynn Margulis, an American evolutionary biologist whose name is synonymous with symbiosis. Margulis was a single mother of two from the South Side district of Chicago, not the typical scientist of 1960s America. The major theories of evolution at that time, at least in the West, reflected the capitalistic culture of the US in the 20th century and were all competition-oriented. Margulis's genius was to stress the importance of symbiotic or cooperative relationships between species. This was the time of the Cold War, and so her theories were seen as rather communist, favouring the ideology of the enemy state, the Soviet Union. Her paper was rejected by an astonishing 15 journals. Eventually, the *Journal of Theoretical Biology* accepted it.

Her theories are now considered to be some of the most important in scientific history.[37] She proposed the now widely accepted idea that every living cell operating inside all multi-cellular life on this planet — from trees and flowers, to humans and animals, mushrooms and seaweed — is made up from two life forms that, billions of years ago, decided to work together. The waste products of one feed the other, and vice versa. Over time, like old married couples, these organisms become so dependent that they couldn't survive without each other.

Margulis is known as the woman who defied Darwin,[38] and yet we don't hear *survival of the most cooperative*. Darwin was a man of his time and place — Victorian Britain. It was one of the most mercenary, cut-throat societies that has ever existed. In that culture, it is no wonder that Darwin's theories were all about survival of the fittest. It comes as no surprise, then, that of the theories on music, Charles Darwin's ideas focus on competition.[39] He suggested that song might have originated before we as a species started to speak (which could certainly be true). He took his cue from birds and suggested that we evolved by singing love songs to each other — I mean, isn't a love song nothing more than an elaborate mating ritual? But then, this dismisses the myriad different calls that birds have: a call that alerts their young to which predators are around and what action to take,[40] calls to claim territory, calls to tell their young how far they are from the nest, along with body language postures. To give birds, and ourselves, just one reason to use song is to do both species a disservice.

Daniel Levitin, author of *This Is Your Brain on Music*,[41] ponders the idea that there might be something in Darwin's sexual selection argument. Let's go along with the idea for a moment.

If you consider that good musicians need time to learn their instruments, this suggests that, unlike the rest of the hunter-gatherers around them, they haven't needed to spend hours looking for food. Being good at music therefore might, at least indirectly, indicate that you are a great hunter. You've had time to learn to play an instrument, after all. Furthermore, consider what makes a good hunter. It's not just being able to accurately shoot an arrow or throw a rock — no, good hunters need to have a creative brain in order to respond to the ever-changing reactions of their prey. Being good at making music is a very clear and direct sign that you are creative and therefore will pass on better genes. Levitin suggests that Mick Jagger, and other rock stars, have managed to sleep with thousands of partners by displaying this.

Levitin suggests that Mick has fathered eight children with five different women — despite the fact that, in his words, 'Mick is no looker'* — because he has displayed his creative prowess to millions. Furthermore, just as birds do, Mick Jagger sings to attract his many lovers, and perhaps song does fulfil this role.

Another theory — from Steven Pinker, a professor of psychology at Massachusetts Institute of Technology and a celebrated populariser of science — which perhaps sums up the bland and reductionist side of Western culture, is that music is simply auditory cheesecake.[42] That is to say, we didn't evolve to like cheesecake, but we did evolve to like fatty and sugary things. Music, like cheesecake, evolved because we like and respond well to some of the things related to it, such as language. It piggybacked on language, which is useful for our survival. We could easily survive without cheesecake, and we could easily live without song. There is another guy, Dan Sperber,[43] who calls music an 'evolutionary parasite'. Imagine those two guys DJing a party — that'd be fun!

It's hard to imagine music's place in culture, as we tend to view it through the eyes of people who have been passive receivers of music. Our modern culture favours a small number of people performing to a disproportionately high number of others. Back in 1997, for example, Jean-Michel Jarre performed for the 850th birthday celebration of Moscow, a concert attended by 3.5 million people. That's more people than there were on the Earth 12,000 years ago![44] And millions more watched on TV, including myself.

This passive form of entertainment, singers and musicians performing without participation, might be

---

* Don't forget that beauty is in the eye of the beholder. I'm not sure everyone, including myself, would agree that Mick is no looker.

a relatively new concept as far as we modern humans are concerned. We can trace the idea back to the fourth century,[45] a time when only singers ordained and trained by the Church were allowed to sing during a Christian service. The rest of the congregation were not considered to be worthy of giving praise. In other cultures, singing remains something to be shared as a group.

It's argued that singing and musical accompaniment started around the late-night fires of our ancestors. Having attended social meets with other foragers for the Association of Foragers, I can attest to the fact that we don't forage at night. For many of this group, the obsession is constant, the search for food never ending. But foragers do not have night vision, and so firelight creates a place where stories, songs, and music are shared. It would have been no different for our Palaeolithic ancestors, and so the advent of music is likely to have really started to take hold around the first fire pits.[46,47] And it would have aided social interactions. Maybe the reason why Neanderthals lived in such small, isolated groups was because shared music never existed for them.[48] The one Neanderthal musical artefact, a bone flute, may possibly be nothing more than a hyena's lunch, after all.[49] Perhaps this shared capacity to make music together and bond in larger groups is another reason why *Homo sapiens* became the dominant species of hominid.

I wanted to explore this notion. I wanted to experience what music meant to me. Drumming felt powerful; I knew it was something that could bring groups together, could put me in touch with my subconscious, and perhaps could help with grieving. What, then, of song — what were the boundaries of song? I thought again about the bonding I felt by singing with friends. I'd not done that in a long time. I thought about how I put the radio on, after cooking three meals a day from scratch has produced another mountain of mess that needs sorting. How it makes the job so much easier. I'd go as far as saying a delight (especially if you combine it with microdosing).

Singing in a group, though, was something that was missing from my life. If it's what secured our place as the dominant ape on the planet, then surely it would be quite a pleasurable activity. I got in touch with local singer Molly King, who hosts wellbeing choirs, and we arranged to meet up.

On the way there, I walked through Barton Hill, the estate we used to live in before we had children. I spent a lot of time going between there and the then more vibrant surrounding estates of St Werburgh's and Easton. We lived there for around six years, and during that time we helped run a co-operative café book shop, had an allotment, and went out drinking. The nearby Lawrence Hill train station was our most used and preferred transport. I sat and wrote my first and second book in that area. It was very familiar territory, albeit from over a decade ago.

As I walked, memories started to flow back. People I hadn't thought about in years, a restaurant that only lasted a month, parties, and all sorts of little moments. I was content, happy, and started nonchalantly singing a tune. Like the memories, I felt like it was something that harked back to this earlier time — it was a tune I hadn't thought about in years. It was like my feet wanted to sing that tune, that it was somehow embedded in the place. I took note of it and continued to walk. As I got into Easton and St

Werburgh's I similarly found myself singing tunes that I felt had been committed to history. Pop songs from the early 2000's, I mean, not even stuff I wanted to share.

For a moment I shuddered at my bad taste, then I consoled myself with the thought that this could have been a way in which people found food. If we all sang in praise of a place where we had found food, that would help us to remember where it was. It's partly why people with Alzheimer's might be able to recall songs;[51] in ancient times, it could literally keep people alive.

I digress: back to Molly and singing as a group activity. We met up in the rather appropriately named Garden of Easton, a cafe on the trendier north-east side of Bristol. I mentioned how when I was working in factories and warehouses, I'd noticed a camaraderie when certain songs came on. How singing together made the day go a little quicker and lightened the mood. I asked her if her wellbeing choirs were a little different. This was her response:

> I think we are really lacking connection in the West. I think that's the big problem, loneliness and not knowing properly how to connect with people. I think singing and music is an ancient way to connect — we've just forgotten how. We've got all this shame around it, because we've got this strange idea of what singing is. Just over the border in Ireland, they don't have that. They sing all the time; it's part of the culture. When you grow up with that, it's just normal and natural, and it just brings joy. One of the first things that people say to me when I tell them I'm a singer is, 'Oh, I can't sing.'

I include myself in this category. I can hear my voice singing along to the radio; I hear the bum notes. I hear the notes I can't reach — I don't celebrate the notes that I do sing well. I then found reassurance in what Molly went on to say:

> It's like a confession, and it's just not true. We are all singers and dancers ... People think you have to be good rather than just seeing it as an expression. We are all trying to be perfectionists; it's hard. I absolutely have a whole load of that myself. I think this is why I like facilitating the group. I can completely get rid of that, I don't have to try and be good when I'm teaching, when I'm just facilitating people to try and express themselves.

Molly invited me to find out for myself. Out of the blue, she told me there was a meeting later that week. That I should come along. I visibly retracted into myself, curled up into a ball on my seat. This wasn't at all what I wanted, I realised. The idea of singing in front of people, and presumably people from the cool side of town who did this all the time, was frankly terrifying.

I left Molly and jumped on the local train home. I'd made my excuses; the class was on a Thursday evening, the same night that one of us had to take our son to taekwondo. I had an out, until Emma said, 'Matt [the instructor] is on holiday this week, and they're not meeting back until next week. You can go singing if you want.' Shit.

I arrived to find a group of mainly younger women and one man. I'd been working on this book, trying to meet the deadline, which was less than a week away. If you have ever written a PhD or a dissertation, got married or done anything that requires a deadline, then you'll understand where my head was at. My thoughts were of little other than writing. I'd apologised to Emma for being boring — I knew I was, but I had to discharge the weight of that deadline somehow. It was coming out in constantly talking about it.

We sat in a circle and went around the room, each given one word to describe how we felt.

Excited, sad, joyful, fizzy ...

It got to me, and I couldn't think of just one word. I gave three: 'in my head'. I was. I felt uptight and nervous; I could feel my smile was false, along with all the other signs of being totally out of my comfort zone. Just as I suspected, I was terrified — what the fuck was I doing here among these real singers?

Then we all closed our eyes and made what Molly called qi gong sounds.[52] Molly told us about how these ancient sounds would help us to get more in tune with our own bodies.[53] I withheld my judgement and joined in. We made six sounds; each, we were told, corresponded to one of our organs. 'Zzz' for the lungs, 'choreee' for the kidneys, 'shoo' for the liver, 'harrr' for the heart, 'whoor' for the spleen, and finally 'heee', which corresponded to the triple warmer that is said to balance our endocrine system.[54] I'm not prepared either to agree with or dismiss these claims; I just don't know enough about qi gong, the fascia,[55] and Chinese medicine. What I will say is that closing my eyes and making these noises as part of a group had an instantaneous effect on me. I was happy and felt like a different person, the relaxed version of me — it was great.

Molly then had us jamming, copying sounds that she

was making, similar to chanting. Chanting is practised in many religions, and it can be another way to enter into an altered state.[56] It is also thought to help people with anxiety, depression, and PTSD symptoms.[57] We didn't chant for long enough to enter an altered state; it felt more playful than the chanting that religious people seem to practise. A grin started to appear on my face at this point, and I don't know if it left.

My comfort zone was to expand a little more that night, as next up Molly had us dancing. To get our blood flowing. When did I last dance in front of anyone but my family without drugs or alcohol? I'm pretty sure it was back when I was 13 and first heard Chicago house music. I can remember telling people I was on drugs so that I could dance like an idiot — this night, I didn't have to. I could just dance like an idiot. The room filled with whoops as everyone skipped around each other. It didn't feel uncomfortable to look at anyone right in their eyes. I felt comfortable with these strangers; it was as if they were old friends. Like the drumming, it felt natural — it felt amazing.

Suitably limbered up, we now returned to a group. Standing in a circle, we were invited to make loops. Molly tapped out a rhythm, and we all kept time with each other. Some weird and funky noises came out of us all. I spent most of my early teen years stoned, and on one particularly memorable occasion three of us made a tune. It came from nowhere; all of us were non-musicians. Yet, we found our place with each other — bass, treble, it was all there. I remember it sounding magical and thought it was some fluke — maybe we were so stoned that it just *sounded* good to us. I thought it would never happen again. But now I was to find out just how natural it is. Everyone in the group held a rhythm, looped their own sounds with each other. I wasn't stoned, not drunk, just my usual straight self. Here we all were in harmony with each other.

There were more exercises, including singing one of Molly's own compositions. I'm sure I missed a few notes here and there, but the performative aspect didn't exist. It didn't matter.

Just as with the drumming, it felt like I'd connected with these strangers. That if I were to bump into anyone in that room again, I could chat to them like a friend. I'm still grinning thinking about that evening. I'm trying to work out how I can get my son to taekwondo and then travel the three miles across town to join the wellbeing choir. Of all the aspects of the New Wild Order, singing like that in a group feels like something I want to be part of my life on a far more regular basis. The connection it brings might just be a fundamental part of what we are missing in Western secular culture.

NEW WILD (YOUR) MUSIC

Community notice boards are a good place to start your search for drumming circles in your local area, as are online groups. I also find simply asking around was helpful too, especially if you ask the right people, so pop into a shop that sells drums!

To find some shamanic beats that appeal to you, find some drummers on YouTube; try out a few before you settle on one. They seem to increase every day, but unfortunately the quantity is greater than the quality. I personally prefer bullroarers and drumming together.

Choirs are popping up all over the place at the moment — again, check notice boards, online groups, and ask around to find yours. If you live in a town or city, you don't have to settle on the first you find. Keep looking until you find one that feels like a good fit. Many offer the first session for free.

If you struggle to find a drumming circle or a choir, consider starting your own.

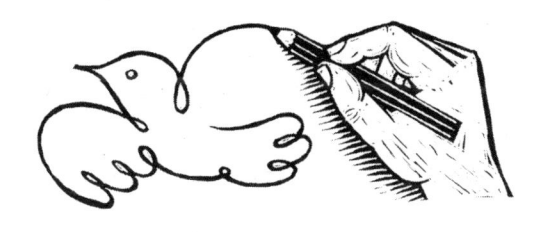

CHAPTER SIX

Art

> *'Art cannot be separated from life. It is the expression of the greatest need of which life is capable, and we value art not because of the skilled product, but because of its revelation of a life's experience.'*
>
> ROBERT HENRI, 1910

I believe that when we create, we need a link with something natural. So that when I, or anyone else, gets to work on any artistic endeavour, be it painting, drawing, writing, singing, acting, dancing or composing music, it becomes something that is an expression of the natural world — and maybe that natural world is more alive than we realise.

Sometimes, as I write, especially poetry and prose, it feels like the forest is breathing through me, Andy Hamilton, a human. You could argue that, on some level at least, the forest* or natural world is actually breathing through us all — I mean, psychically there is an interchange going on, after all. We breathe in all the substances that the trees use to defend themselves and communicate with each other,[1] and the trees use the carbon dioxide that we breathe out to help them grow.[2] Also, whether we like it or not, we are utterly dependent on the natural world for all our resources. Right now, you might be in a building, on a train, in a car or any other man-made environment. Look around you and count the things you see that come from within ten miles (16 kilometres) of where you sit. I don't mean from a nearby shop, I mean look at the plastic, wood, glass, and metal that make up the objects that surround you. Where did it all come from? I'd be shocked if you knew; I've no idea where any of the parts that make up this pen I'm writing with came from, nor the paper that I'm writing on, and even less of a clue where the parts of the computer I'll type this up on come from.

We may live without ever witnessing, let alone taking part in, our clothes being made, our food being grown, our houses being built or the resources for our phones being mined, processed, and manufactured. So of course we feel a bit detached.

In a more connected society, we might experience the world differently. Perhaps we'd even start to treat the natural world like a family member, as our ancestors did. These were people who survived day to day using the resources in their local area and the things that lived in it. The year in which I ate a piece of wild food every day from the same valley made

---

* I use the term 'forest' here to indicate the untamed, wild world rather than an actual forest.

me see the world differently. I not only became part of the area, I was that area; the minerals and phytonutrients (plant nutrients) became my blood, bones, and organs. Whenever I walked to that spot, I felt a profound sense of belonging.

In this context, the idea that all living things have a consciousness, the notion that there is something of the spiritual essence inside all living things, that everything has a soul, becomes clearer. Imagine that feeling amplified, imagine knowing the nettle patch your shirt came from, the patch the deer you eat favour, the spring you always drink from. Real or imagined, you would start to feel very differently about the place you called home. If you, too, had to rely on your local area for everything, it would become your favourite restaurant, clothes shop, pub, and maybe even place of worship all in one. Imagine the love you might feel for those places all rolled together. Something of this idea still remains, and we still have holy or sacred rivers, such as the Ganges in India, the Saru in Japan, the Zuñi in the US, and the Niger in Africa.

It is no wonder, then, that the idea of everything having a soul was once universal. This idea is known as animism, an academic catch-all term used to encompass a wide variety of belief systems that have this concept at their core; it comes from the Latin word *anima*, meaning breath, spirit or life.

It's a mode of spiritual belief that can be found from Asia,[3] to Africa,[4] to Oceania,[5] and across the Americas,[6] the assumption being that we were all animists once.[7] That is, according to Rupert Sheldrake, the biochemist and author, the only exception to this belief is our own culture — post-industrial Western culture.[8]

The ubiquitous nature of animism suggests that

traditional art and practices might be embedded firmly within human culture and land. When I watch the birds in our garden grabbing feathers, twigs, and fluff from the tumble drier in our neighbours' shed, I wonder if their nests are totally functional or if there is some artistry to them. Consider the Australian bowerbird, after all — it's almost indisputable that their ground nests, or bowers, are anything but a work of art.[9] They place nuts, flowers, can rings, snail shells, and anything they seem to find beautiful around their intricately made bowers in order to attract a mate.

It's of no surprise, then, that art pre-dates modern humans, and the oldest piece of art found is thought to be a freshwater clam shell with a zig-zag line etched into it. It's half a million years old, and therefore pre-dates *Homo sapiens*, modern humans. It was found at Trinil, Indonesia,[10] in the 1890s by Dutch geologist Eugène Dubois. It was possibly worn as decoration by *Homo erectus*, a species of archaic human from the Pleistocene, who first walked this earth two million years ago.

I'd love to report that art then took off, that *Homo erectus* quickly progressed from making scratches on shells, that archaeologists have unearthed a Pleistocene version of the Louvre. I can't. Truth is, we don't know. It might have been that *Homo erectus* would make temporary sculptures by piling branches onto each other, or that they weaved grass to make exquisite dolls, all items that would disintegrate without a trace. I've heard it said that archaeology is like standing in a room with a locked door, staring through the keyhole to see what is going on two rooms away.

However, there is some evidence that is noteworthy. Circles in the sand that are over 135,000 years old have been found perfectly preserved as sandstone, and they could be considered art.[11] Perhaps the artist was displaying the notion that our actions can ripple through time. Further back in time, but more controversially, *Homo naledi* — an ancient cousin of *Homo sapiens* — may have scratched a cross-hatch pattern onto the rock at a place where bodies were found, suggesting it was somewhere that may have had some spiritual significance.[12] This was between 241,000 and 350,000 years ago; however, talk about this in some circles, and you'll suddenly see mild-mannered academics get quite hot under the collar, as interpretation of these findings' significance remains as contentious as pineapple on a pizza. So, the most compelling and most agreed-upon artefact of ancient art seems to be a rock with a cross-hatch pattern painted on using ochre.[13] It was painted around 73,000 years ago.

It's entirely possible that our ancestors or the living things around us experience the world differently to us. Perhaps living things do all have a consciousness, and perhaps they don't see a separation between nature and humanity, just as our ancestors didn't. Or maybe our ancestors just liked drawing on caves — we may never know.

If our ancestors did believe that everything has a consciousness, and there is no clear boundary between animals and humans, how would that have expressed itself? Would this be an explanation for the lion man unearthed in a cave in southern Germany? It, or perhaps he, has a human body and stands tall like a human, but has a lion's head. This is the 40,000-year-old, 30-centimetre-tall figure of a lion man[14] carved from a mammoth's tusk. He must have had some significance to the people who encountered him, as he has been worn down by multiple human hands. It begs the question: why a lion man? Could it be that the original artist wanted to convey a feeling that they were aware of a consciousness which matched or even rivalled human consciousness? That perhaps they saw little separation between the human and the animal?

Were he a lone figure, we might dismiss this notion, and yet we were still making human lion sculptures in 500 BCE.[15] Time and time again, these part-human, part-animal figures appear: we have the Alkonost bird people of Russia;[16] the half-snake, half-woman Echidna of ancient Greece;[17] Anansi, the half-man, half-spider originating from Ghana;[18] and, just recently dated to be the earliest piece of narrative art (at the time of writing), the 51,200-year-old half-pig, half-human figure from Leang Karampuang on Sulawesi, Indonesia.[19]

Part of me wonders whether these representations were made by ancient childminders, whether this lion man was simply used to illustrate a story passed down through generations to entertain a gaggle of wild children. After all, a version of animism still lives on, and children's literature is full of talking animals, fruit, vegetables,[20] and pots.[21]

Archaeological evidence of these first works of art might only tell part of the story and, in order to understand how humans might have thought, we have to look at recent groups of people who hold animist cultural beliefs. The Sámi, for example. They are a people who live in the Sápmi region,* a land mass that stretches across northern parts of Norway, Sweden, Finland, and the Kola Peninsula in Russia. In living memory, these people were nomadic, travelling

---

* Once referred to as Lapland.

with their herds of reindeer — indeed, there still are herders, although many now use motorised sleds. In such an inhospitable region, they were utterly dependent on these animals. Not just for their meat, but for their skins to make clothes and bladders for carrying water, and their bones to make tools. They would talk to their reindeer or sing songs, known as joiks, when they herded them,[22] and they made artworks honouring them.[23]

It's perhaps hard for us to fully understand this way of life: farming and, more essentially, trading with those who live in alien lands, lands that we may never set foot in. Feeding, clothing, and surrounding ourselves with things from faraway places means the link with the natural world around us is severed; we do not experience it with quite the same intimacy or spiritual reverence. For the Sámi, it would be very important to ensure that the next generation felt the same reverence for the animals that supplied their food, shelter, and tools. Indeed, our early ancestors would all have had to have a working knowledge of the animals they used for food, and the animals that used them for food. Stories are always great vessels for information that flows down through the ages, and perhaps stories about lion men, pig people, and human-bird hybrids all needed some illustration. Art may, then, have originated as a way to stop children from being eaten by lions.

But is art quite so important to us today? Maybe so. According to the Mayo Clinic, people who take up creative activities in middle age are less likely to suffer from memory loss and mild cognitive impairment.[24] When we create, we help to stop old neurons from dying and support the growth of new ones. Simply put: use it or lose it. I'm turning 50 soon and wondered if this was why I found myself naturally *drawn* towards artistic endeavours, something that I haven't really engaged with for years.

I used to blame my early conditioning (my upbringing), but there is only so long you can use that as a defence. I'm like two in every 250 people: I'm a monozygotic identical twin.[25] We were born at a time before ultrasound was the norm, and our parents didn't know there would be two of us until my brother decided to join us. As infants and right up until our teenage years, we looked very alike; there are some photos where I don't even know which one I am, so what hope did anyone else have? Even our mum used to dress us in different colours to tell us apart. As we grew and went to school, I'd get called the boring twin, or the good (as in, goody-goody) twin. In fact, I remember being the lonely twin.

Teachers would make us read together, or play the same part in the school play — sometimes at the same time. We'd be referred to as 'the twins'. It wasn't a good grounding for a harmonious adult relationship. As we aged, it felt like we were playing out Freud's theory of the narcissism of small differences,[26] the idea that feuds and ridicule are highly likely when you are more alike — and we battled. We, or at least I, are hyper-aware of the small differences, and sometimes that would wind me up to the point of distraction. I can never understand why my brother doesn't do things right — the way I do! As we've grown older, we've grown more alike in some ways, our jobs are very similar,* and as such, the feuds have grown, and we've drifted apart.

We were a bit more harmonious as children. I strove

---

* If you ever want to read a book on wild ruins, he's your man.

for my individuality, to be recognised as different, even at the cost of things I enjoyed. I loved drawing and painting as a child, but I was never quite as good as him. He had the ability to sit and concentrate on a drawing, and I wanted it to be great straight away and so just stopped. What was the point if I was never going to be as good as him? But can I truly put that at my brother's door as, maybe, what was true for me was true for everyone?

Perhaps I didn't apply myself because that is a little bit terrifying. Julia Cameron, author of the international bestseller *The Artist's Way*,[27] states that choosing to be more creatively focused can be disturbing — that we see an artistic life as all or nothing and therefore fail to pursue it at all.

I'd have done well to read a little of Kurt Vonnegut; it might've released me from the idea of having to be any good before I even tried. I might not have waited until I was approaching the autumn of my life before I made any kind of mark on a canvas, for Vonnegut states that it doesn't matter how badly you practise art, you should just do it anyway, as it makes your soul grow.

The soul can be a tricky subject, with neuroscience suggesting that all functions can be attributed to the brain — something I find rather inhuman.[28] Still, what can't be denied is that practising artistic endeavours can be a powerful therapeutic tool. I've experienced it helping to address historical and current trauma. A Ghanaian musician I once knew sang to his family of the grief he felt after the loss of his unborn child. He had a host of songs that connected his family to both positive and negative life events. Counsellor (and Cowichan) Lyla Harman recognises, too, the power of art, and she integrates painting, songs, knitting, basket weaving, and even songs into her practice.[29]

Writer Terry Sullivan talks of how it has helped him. In 1993 he was dozing off on an evening train. He awoke, abruptly, to the sight of panicked passengers running away from a gunman.[30] The gunman was firing on the other passengers. Terry managed to hide and escape, despite at one point making eye contact with the gunman. Six people died on that train that evening, with a further 19 seriously injured. The incident shook him, and depression and a series of nightmares followed. He felt he couldn't articulate his feelings. Instead, he took to creating an artwork that he called *Before-the-Dawn Perspective*,[31] a rather haunting piece with empty train seats and mismatched images of a revolver. He suggests that creating this image helped to display his feelings.

Terry asked professor of psychiatry Dr Robert Ursano if creating his work could have helped him to find meaning in the incident, Ursano agreed that putting the elements together and then putting them to rest would have helped. He also suggested that traumatised people will often choose to write down their problems, and that any form of expression that you are comfortable with is just as valid.

I know that after my friend Doug died when I was 17 (see Chapter Two), I struggled to find any outlet for the traumatic feelings I needed to express. Yet I felt a compulsion to create something, anything. I started to think about painting, but I didn't believe I had any of the talent or the tools to do it. Instead, I picked up a wad of A4 paper and a biro. Over the next few weeks, I created a comic book that I called *A Ropey Mess of Shit* — the title was an attempt to excuse myself from the naivety of the text and the drawing. I was highly self-critical of the work. I think I eventually destroyed it.

Yet, in hindsight I was doing just as Terry did. I'd found a way to express the feelings that I was struggling to articulate in any other way. The comic book depicted the night we were chased by the man who struck Douglas, his funeral, and the time I spent down in Cornwall. Everything that I was processing at the time. Both Terry and I had stumbled across art therapy.

The interdisciplinary study of art and psychology began in the US in the 1940s, when Margaret Naumburg started publishing clinical cases of her new practice.[32] She, and others, were finding new ways for soldiers traumatised by the World Wars to express themselves. It wasn't always possible for them to articulate what was going on, as trauma can affect the speech centres,[33] thus making speaking therapies rather pointless.

I wondered, then, if perhaps the impetus behind some prehistoric art was similar. If there was any link between a proliferation of cave art and an ancient traumatic event. It turns out that there was: around 42,000 years ago, there was an event that is now known as the Adams event,[34] or the Laschamp event.[35] What happened was a short reversal of the Earth's magnetic field — some call it a polar flip — the transition lasted for 250 years and the poles stayed reversed for another 440 years. During the transition, the magnetic field around the Earth decreased to around 5 per cent of what it is now, and it only increased to 25 per cent of where our field currently stands when the poles were switched.

It didn't affect every region in the same way; the worst of the problems hit Europe and Oceania. This would have done more than just mess up your compass. It resulted in more cosmic rays hitting the Earth, which meant a large increase in charged particles from the sun reaching Earth — these are cancer-causing ultraviolet particles. Lightning storms raged, the ozone layer was destroyed,[36] and the weather was as erratic as a hyperactive toddler after a party. The knock-on effect is thought to have been catastrophic for the mega-fauna of Oceania, and countless extinctions followed. It may also have ushered in the demise of the Neanderthals.[37]

What this must have been like to live through is anybody's guess, yet I think there can be little dispute that it would have been rather traumatic. Humans, however, had a secret weapon in naturally occurring ochre. It's a pigment that is still used today by the Himba people of Namibia, who mix it with butterfat to make otjize, a substance that is used as suntan lotion. This would have helped to protect them from the harsh sun, giving them an advantage when gathering food. Ochre is also the pigment that is used in cave art. Considering the explosion of cave art across the planet around the time of the Adams event,[38] did our ancient ancestors feel a compulsion to express their emotions on the walls of their caves? If so, art therapy might be a lot older than was once thought.

Writing is another form of art therapy that will help those dealing with traumatic thoughts and feelings related to a stressful event. In various studies, expressive writing for 20 minutes or more over several sessions has been linked to a number of positive health outcomes.[39] It's been seen to help reduce blood pressure,[40] pain for patients suffering from rheumatoid arthritis,[41] and depressive symptoms.[42]

During my last flare-up of my autoimmune condition

— minimal change disease — when I had to take steroids again, I drew in combination with writing, and for the first time in over a decade I didn't feel quite so insane, something I feel every time I have to take them. I'd managed the condition differently. I continued the writing with some drawing. Combining the two mediums, I found, kept my mind away from the effects of the pills.

The frequent practice of drawing or painting was starting to pay off. I'd been pondering over an old friend called George. George was one of those people who just seemed to be brilliant at everything, and charismatic to boot. He decided he wanted to act, wrote a play and starred in it, and it was good. He picked up the saxophone, and within a week he was pottering about playing it like he had done for years. George also started to draw — horses, mostly — and they were, of course, perfect. George was self-assured, and I pondered whether perhaps that was all it would take to switch mindset. That I could drop what was holding me back. After all, I had the same DNA as someone else who could draw.

I started with a biro and a notepad, sat in the shed on the allotment, and drew what I saw. I carried the notepad around and continued this process, daily at one point, upgrading to watercolours and then taking a few — no more than six — classes. I'd paint natural landscapes, and love drawing or painting trees and clouds. What I found fascinating was just how quickly I changed from feeling like I couldn't draw to capturing something of the world around me. After a year, I felt proud enough of my work to exhibit in a local arts trail. I'd developed a style and had themes, things that proper artists do.

Proust also suggests that adults and our habits can get in the way of appreciating the world, that we don't spend time revelling in the everyday. The major difference in my world that I noticed after undertaking an artistic practice is that I appreciate the sky more. There seems to be more drama, more colour, more beauty up there than anywhere else that I look. I decided to concentrate on painting clouds and have subsequently fallen in love with them, finding an appreciation, far beyond what I thought possible, for the work of Monet, Constable, Van Gogh, Scottish artist James Morrison, and of course Turner — cloud painters that seem to capture the spirit in the skies and, with that, something of themselves, too.

Human beings have always had ways to express themselves, through storytelling, art, dance, and song. However, the fact remains that many of us don't. The very act of creating seems to be something we leave behind while we are still at school. In the US, around half of all adults did not create or perform any art in a 12-month period.[43] Worse, if you posed the question 'Would you describe yourself as creative?' and asked five industrial nations, Germany, the USA, the UK, France, and Japan, only 41 per cent of people would respond positively. It would appear, too, that those over the age of 75 are least likely to engage in the arts, with a massive 36 per cent not engaging at all, compared to 19 per cent of all other age groups.[44]

The fact that 36 per cent of over-75s do not engage with the arts is somewhat alarming considering our ageing global population — a population that is expected to reach 9.8 billion by 2050.[45] Of this massive population, it's estimated that one in six of us will be over 65,[46] and around 1.5 billion people will be over 80. The likelihood of getting dementia increases as we age,[47] and considering that dementia already costs 1 per cent of global domestic product, we are heading for a financial and emotional disaster.

Art might do something to mitigate this. As part of the process of making art a habit, I joined a creative meet-up group run by a local artists' studio and community enterprise.[48] The ages of the participants varied, but the majority were over the age of 65. It's a great group of people, and conversations can vary; they have included life after death, growing cannabis, and the sorry state of the number 36 bus. Considering that social isolation can increase the risk of dementia by 50 per cent,[49] simple groups like this weekly session can start to really make a difference to people's lives.

To have overcome my perceived inability to draw has done much for me. It's deepened my appreciation of the natural world, especially the sky, and it's given me something I can sit and join in doing with my children. It's also given me another tool in the box to work through problems. To sit and paint or draw, to study the clouds above my head, is to take me out of myself. To give me fresh eyes with which to view the world.

Proust suggests that we should look at the world with the same generosity as an artist does,[50] and developing an artistic practice does this. It's like a meditation for me — I get excited when I see the way a shaft of light hits a rooftop on one of the houses I can see from my kitchen window. Right now, I'm watching a long branch of hazel bob up and down in the wind. It reminds me of my son when he was a toddler, the way he'd constantly move, and it pleases me to see this. Am I seeing the same spirit that inhabited him back then? I'm not sure, to be honest, and I don't think it really matters. What I do know is that it stirs something in me, and right now I'm grinning while I contemplate it.

So, go on, glance up from this page, and look for something, anything — an object, the sky, a person, your cat. Now really look at it, study it. Watch how the light shines on it; look at the shape of it, and how the world around it interacts with it. Or listen to the way the wind blows through the leaves in the trees around you, or maybe just feel your own bodily sensations. You don't even have to draw, paint or create anything to do all this. How do you feel once you've done that — a little more alive? A little less in your own head?

Hopefully you do, because, I think, if you experience the world in this way, it's hard to feel anything but glad to be alive.

NEW WILD YOUR ARTISTIC PRACTICE

Spend time just passively looking at something wild: a cloud, a tree, a house plant or your partner. Keep looking at it and admire it for its beauty and uniqueness. Imagine that this living thing is doing the same right back at you. My personal favourite is to do this with the sky. So many different colours and expressions exist up there from the moonless night skies, grey overcast days, clouds with purple tints, and huge fluffy clouds that look like great canyons of the sky.

Sometimes we need motivation to get painting or drawing; search community noticeboards for art classes and clubs and join in.

Carry a little notebook around with you and sketch when you get the chance. Talk to artists, ask them about how they view the world. If you have children in your life, especially ones below ten, talk to them about clouds, trees, and plants.

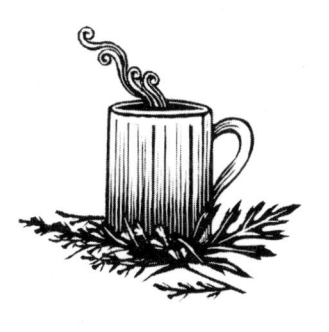

CHAPTER SEVEN

Sleep

'Yes: I am a dreamer. For a dreamer is one who can only find his way by moonlight, and his punishment is that he sees the dawn before the rest of the world.'

OSCAR WILDE, 1891

Next time you can't sleep, take some comfort in knowing that you are not alone — up to half the population of the developed world will suffer from insomnia at some point in their lives. With figures that high, perhaps this is a normal state of affairs for human beings, nothing to worry about. Maybe we have always struggled a little with sleep — could it be a trade-off for having such big brains?

We might look at the last remaining hunter-gatherers for answers — if they too struggle, then the chances are it is a symptom of evolution. Perhaps we used to need someone in our group to stay awake, spear at the ready to defend against a sabre-toothed tiger attack. Yet, neither the Hadza of Tanzania nor the San of Namibia have a word for insomnia. These remaining hunter-gatherer tribes have an average rate of 2 per cent insomnia within their groups,[1] or, in other words, it's small enough not to really be a problem.

The Hadza do sleep a little differently, however: they don't aim for a straight eight hours. In fact, their habits are quite appealing, as they sleep for an average of 6.25 hours a night but make up for it with an opportunistic naptime.[2] Bosses, take note — you might have a better-rested and more productive staff if you decreased the working day and offered breakout rooms complete with hammocks.

If we can assume that the hunter-gatherers slept well before the world *developed*, it wouldn't be too much of a stretch to suggest that insomnia might be a symptom of the artificial environment we have created since the Industrial Revolution. What, then, did our sleep look like in the days before electric light? An experiment by 90s psychiatrist Thomas Wehr suggests that if people are plunged into 14 hours of darkness, as in pre-industrial times, within four weeks we naturally revert to a two-sleep system comprising two four-hour sleeps.[3]

I once found myself naturally falling into this segmented sleep pattern, too; that is to say, two sleeps. I was using a lot of social media and, as such, my middle-of-the-night insomnia was acute, and I found myself lying in bed staring at the ceiling most nights. It went on for weeks, and I felt drained and exhausted. In the end, and in desperation, I just stopped fighting it and got up whenever I awoke. I took to walking the local area at 4.00 am to observe the wildlife. I started to learn some of the constellations, too; they were so clear in the starlit winter sky.

Within a couple of nights, I noticed a change, a shift in my being. Of course, I decided it was a shift back to something primal, animal even. Well, it was at least a refreshing change from the busy head I'd grown used to living with. It was a very welcome state, as it was a calmer process, no room for anxiety or paranoid thoughts. I started to feel that I was a little more in tune with my surroundings, too. At once point, it was as if I could feel beyond my body, as if I was surrounded by a new sense.

I wanted and even believed that I was ridding myself of the old me and replacing him with a 'real' me, and I wanted to believe that I'd personally discovered a new kind of sleep. I can, after all, be prone to such grandiose thinking. Read a few author-written book blurbs, and you'll soon see that most authors have these moments. It's maybe these moments that make us believe we can finish a book. Still, I digress. I knew, at least, that what I felt was beyond my everyday experience. Thankfully, while reading *Dark Skies* by Tiffany Francis-Baker, I found a cure for my delusions of grandeur when I found a reference to the physiological phenomenon that was occurring. Much to my chagrin, it wasn't due to some primeval gene switch, and it certainly wasn't new.

I discovered that, by having two periods of sleep, my levels of prolactin were increasing. Prolactin, meaning 'promote milk', is a luteotropic hormone (LTH) with around 300 functions, chief among them being to aid rest, lower levels of testosterone, help to repair myelin (the fatty substance that surrounds nerve cells), and increase milk production for lactating mothers — something true in 85 per cent of mammals. The latter may come as some consolation for nursing mothers battling with fragmented sleep patterns; you might be so sleep deprived that you can hardly speak, but at least it is helping to keep baby well fed!

Segmented sleep may well have been the norm far more recently than I first thought, too. Reputedly, we were still having two sleeps right up until the Industrial Revolution. According to a 16-year study of literature by historian Roger Ekirch of Virginia Tech, there were over 500 references in diaries, court records, and medical books to first and second sleeps; he even found that the Tiv of central Nigeria still practise this more forgiving way of sleeping. We can still find traces of biphasic sleep patterns in certain cultures — the Spanish siesta, deriving from the Latin phrase *hora sexta*, or 'the sixth hour', is perhaps the most famous example,[4] but we can find similar in China, Italy, and Japan, each with a culturally significant 'nap'.

The Industrial Revolution may have put a stop to biphasic or segmented sleep, but it also had a detrimental impact on our monophasic sleep — our single sleep patterns. The Industrial Revolution didn't just take us out of the country and into the factories and mills of the cities, it bathed us in artificial light and forced us indoors, both of which were disastrously toxic to our natural circadian rhythm — our day–night system.

The majority of us not only work indoors, but we spend our evenings indoors, too, much of the time bathed in artificial light. Not good news for the bleary-eyed among us, as, according to a 2010 study published in the *Journal of Biological Rhythms*,[5] we need six hours a day of bright light (daylight) exposure in order to reduce cortisol levels by 25 per cent. Furthermore, Professor Matthew Walker, sleep specialist and author of *Why We Sleep*, suggests we need this much natural sunlight in order to feel fully awake. This amount of sun would give our circadian rhythm — our natural sleep-and-wakefulness rhythm — the daytime peak it needs to be fully awake, implying that we are sleepwalking throughout our daily lives!

We need to spend 42 hours a week outdoors — that's a quarter of our lives — in order to hit this target. Worldwide, we are very far off this target; according to a US study of 12,000 adults and children, less than 7 per cent of adults spend more than 21 hours outdoors,[6] and the figure across the world suggests much the same.

When I'm writing, I can spend a lot of time indoors, and I've been looking at ways in which to reverse that trend. Walking the kids to school and shopping locally for smaller amounts are two small fixes that, when added together, can total an extra two hours of outdoor time a day, especially when I get up a little bit earlier and take the kids for an extra morning play in the park. I also take tea breaks on my doorstep, we have as many dinners as possible around the garden table, and we often go for a family stroll just around the neighbourhood after we've eaten. I've also taken to working outside with a notepad whenever I can.

Your life might offer different opportunities. Use your imagination, just aim for something enjoyable that you can fit into a routine. I understand that switching behaviour can be difficult; it took me ten years and multiple attempts to quit smoking, for example. However, consider the notion that the brain does prefer new routines over old,[7] so old habits can die easily. Also, in my experience, spending time outdoors can create a positive feedback loop; once you start spending more time outside, you will sleep better and have more energy, making it easier to want to go outside more.

But hey, getting more daylight is only half the battle. We are designed to get a load of darkness, too; you may also find you are dark deprived in the hours before going to sleep. I often tell people, when out in the dark, that ours is a world that never gets properly dark. Next time you are out in a town or city at night, don't go for the light on your phone or a torch. Instead, let your eyes adjust, and you'll see what I mean. Even on moonlit nights in the countryside, you'll often find enough light to walk freely — just perhaps be a little more careful where you tread.

Moreover, we tend to bathe ourselves in light whenever we are inside. This is especially true for those of you who have bright lights on in the house blazing away during the evening, or have to work evenings in brightly lit shops or restaurants. Couple this with the ubiquitous habit of checking your phone, and you are in for some sleep trouble.

I get that phones are highly addictive and difficult to turn off. This is why I switched to an old Nokia phone and have never looked back. Extreme, I know; you could also buy a safe with a timer on it and whack your phone in there at some point in the early evening. It might be enough to break the habit should you want to. It could be worth it if you are suffering from lack of sleep. Dr Dan Siegel[8], clinical professor of psychiatry at UCLA's School of Medicine, suggests that looking at your phone tells the brain not to secrete melatonin. In other words, your phone is telling your brain not to go to sleep yet. Incidentally, research by Kenji Obayashi[9] suggests, too, that ensuring we have appropriate darkness levels in our bedrooms could be a viable preventative tool against depression.

To simulate a time with pre-industrial levels of light, early one May a few years ago, I turned off the gas and electricity at the meter and didn't switch them back on again for another week. The challenge had been set by a magazine editor, and she insisted that I didn't use telecommunications or any motorised transport, either. I cycled everywhere, including a 100-mile (160-kilometre) round trip to the next big city; I collected wood and lit a fire not only to cook on, but to heat up all the hot water I needed for washing. At night I used a single beeswax candle to illuminate the living room. What I found was that I started getting up with the birds and going to bed when the sun went down at around 9.00 pm. It wasn't just that I got bored with no TV to watch or radio to listen to — after all, I could read and keep my diary up to date by candlelight. It was because by 9.00 pm I found myself unable to keep my eyes open, and I slept more soundly than I had done in years.

Subsequently, I've used this experience to help my family and their sleep health, not to the same extreme but a watered-down, realistic version that fits in with our lifestyle. My kids sleep with the curtains open, a happy accident due to my suspect DIY skills and *I'll do it tomorrow* attitude, and my son's tendency to swing on all that he finds. Whatever the original cause, they seem to prefer it that way. By spring, there is enough light at bedtime for them to read for a bit. They are allowed to read or quietly play for as long as they like on the proviso that they won't turn on the lights. I find that by time the sun has fully gone down, they are both fast asleep; on occasion, we have to carry bodies from the middle of the floor back into bed, but otherwise they even take themselves to bed. I must note that I fully intend to fix the curtain rail by summer, as last year they stayed up far too late too often!

Downstairs, we swap the main light for lamps in the living room and ensure no other light is on. I'd like to say we swap the TV for music, but we don't every night. What I am rigid about is turning off my computer. On the nights that I don't follow this routine, mainly if I'm checking for something that could easily wait until the morning, I don't sleep well.

It's not just since having children that I have started to appreciate a good night's sleep above most things in life. Nothing can quite prepare you for the onslaught of early mornings, night-time dramas, and sheer exhaustion that goes with having children. When my son was two, I even had a series of tests to find out why I was so fatigued. It turned out I wasn't a celiac, my iron level was fine, and I didn't have cancer or any other life-threatening diseases; I was just really, really tired, with a touch of hypochondria.

Nevertheless, the lack of sleep affected much of my waking life, and it's not been until my kids have got older and I've started to get more sleep that I'm starting to see a lowering of my blood pressure, some weight loss, and my anxiety and depression levels decreasing, and I am generally feeling more human again.

It's a woe shared by new parents across the world — and if you are a new parent reading this, you might want to skip to the next paragraph now, as news that you are in for a long haul might not go down too well. A study published in the journal *Sleep* suggests that sleep doesn't really return to normal levels until the kids are around four to six years old.[10] I'd agree with this data, with the added caveat that they will still have bad dreams or just get up in the night and want to come in with you. I'm also sure that the teenage years will come with their own set of sleep-related challenges.

Over the last three years or more, I've got into the practice of asking myself a question before I go to sleep, thinking about what is puzzling me then trusting my dreams to give me some insight. Sometimes, I don't have to go to sleep with that intention, I just awake with the solution to a problem. It feels like a regular session of psychotherapy, a way to keep in touch with things that eat away at me on a subconscious level.

This morning, for example, I was wondering how to deal with someone who feels emotionally stuck in the past — let's call them Terry. Terry is always reliving old events and holding on to the pain they caused, and subsequently getting angry. I dreamed I was the captain of a ship — I was a middle-aged woman, for some reason. I was, reluctantly, picking up an award for my brilliance. Along came a group of naked protestors. I walked up to them and said, 'No,' and they backed off. I then said, 'Is there any one of you who will talk sensibly?' A small child emerged, and we started negotiating. I knew then that I had to approach the hurt child Terry and not the angry adult Terry if we were going to move forward. The award was due to the fact that I've another book coming out soon, and I knew that Terry would find that difficult, that jealousy would rear its head. I had to ensure that I didn't bring it up in front of Terry, and shy away from anything that might be seen as *showing off*. I felt that I had a strategy to work with, and the weight of the problem lightened a little.

The details of a dream can easily be missed, and sometimes that's where the most important messages are. It can take a bit of training to recall them. Author of *Why We Dream*, Alice Robb, talks of how she has kept a dream journal for most of her adult life.[11] She focuses through the haze of a dream and looks for a detail. This helps her to find the rest of the narrative in the dream; once she does, she can often pull together the rest of it so she can write it down. Over time, her journal entries have got more detailed and longer.

You need not record every dream you have. I find it's not always possible; family commitments, alarms going off for work, having a partner next to you who would rather go back to sleep cuddling you than have you putting the lights on and scribbling in a *little fucking notebook again*. But it is worth trying to record the more important ones, the ones that stand out. That way, it's easier to tolerate, too.

Dreams can influence more than just how we deal with emotional problems. Some authors have had dreams influence them, too: Lewis Carroll got the inspiration for 'Jabberwocky' from a dream,[12] while Stephen King transcribes his dreams directly to free him from writer's block,[13] an action that owes some credit to Mary Shelley,[14] who, while sheltering from a storm in Geneva with Percy Shelley and Lord Byron, wrote down what she described as 'a waking dream' that was later to become her classic novel, *Frankenstein*. Graham Greene really ran with this idea, and much of his work was influenced by his dreams.[15] His mistress stated that he would write in the morning and read just before bed, thus allowing his subconscious to work on re-drafts in the night.

I find an interaction with my own dreams is something that keeps me feeling balanced. They can also be a powerful tool to help my creative flow.

I don't just interact with dreams; over the last few years, I've started having visions, too. My friend Ray, the beer-writing guy, is quite worried. Although I do sometimes question my own sanity, I am personally pretty comfortable with this state of being. You see, visions don't quite fit into the modern world. They can't easily be explained. Anil Seth, a professor of cognitive and computational neuroscience at the University of Sussex, can help.[16] He suggests that our brain often fills in the gaps, that we have some kind of expectation of what we might see based on previous experience. My visions, hallucinations, or whatever you want to call them, often come after I've been engaging with my dreams, drinking more mugwort tea, drumming, meditating or microdosing mushrooms. Not necessarily when I'm directly affected by any of these things, but within a week of tripping or heavy meditation.

For example, the episode with the goddess that I mentioned in the utiseta chapter happened shortly after I'd spent some time microdosing. Some might refer to it as a flashback. I prefer to think that my brain has been engaged in hallucinating and so it makes up the differences. I might see a flash of sunlight reflecting from a window and, as it's opened, it appears to move. Someone making a video call without headphones in the distance, and I hear a voice.* My brain fills in the gaps.

---

* Which should be a hanging offence, along with public TikTok use.

I'm not sure how this works in others but, in the case of Richard Bach, the author of *Jonathan Livingston Seagull*, his 'disembodied voice' made him a lot of money. It gave him the title for his bestselling work. Once he had the title, he set to work and wrote half of it. Eight years passed following the original concept; that was, until he dreamed the entire second half, which enabled him to finish his book.[17]

Something similar happened with this book. A few years ago, I had a very odd feeling, like I had walked into a cave near the office I was renting a mile from my home. It was as real as a vivid dream; I was experiencing the outside world along with this dream state. The cave existed on the edge of my imagination, and I had no real control over it, only what I did in it. I went to the back of the cave, and there was a chest. I had a choice: to walk away or to open the chest and see what was inside. I'm a curious fellow, and so I opened it. Without warning, I was hit by a sadness, one that just hung around. It was a profound melancholy that didn't leave.

I'd wake up every morning feeling like I was grieving, although I really didn't have any reason to grieve, nor did I know who or what I was grieving for. I now believe it was partly due to some of the grief I had pushed away when I lost a friend to suicide, and it happened shortly after hearing of another old school friend, whom I'd not seen in years, who was beaten to death in what was probably a racist attack. I can feel sadness as I write about them, but no longer that raw feeling of grief. Nor do my emotions feel locked away any longer; it feels right to have this low-level sadness about them both. But there were other emotions, too, that I was dealing with — I was also grieving the loss of my youth. I'd got to the point where I knew I was no longer young enough to have a bright future, and this was probably it for me. The level I'd reach.

I didn't fight it. The emotions came out of the chest, and I sat with them. Some clarity formed, and I got to work changing small but significant aspects of my life, looking inside at other memories I'd locked away, working on them. I read some of Marcus Aurelius — the Stoic philosopher — the *Tao Te Ching*, Michel de Montaigne, and more — in fact, anything I could get my hands on that might help, absorbing their wisdom as best I could. I did have an idea to write a book that I wanted to call *Fully Functioning Human*, which summed up my quest at the time, but really I was just getting well.

Then, one morning, while sitting at my desk alone, I saw the words 'New Wild Order' float past. I knew I had to grab them. Later that day, I was out walking, and when I went past the point where I'd felt the cave, it was back. I felt I'd left it and was closing the chest behind me. The depression lifted, and I felt I was ready to take on the world. I had a new confidence and energy. I knew these words — New Wild Order — had power, power perhaps to transform me. The ideas slowly formed and, over time, I put together an outline to write this book — a book that has been heavily influenced by the worlds that live just beyond.

I realised, too, that healing just takes time. Dr Mary Z. McCullough suggests that 'we heal at the speed of nature'.[18] I couldn't have put it more succinctly myself. I think perhaps that is what I've learned more than anything through this process. That none of us is perfect, we are all muddling through, and that perhaps our society is far more broken than we are. Mental health could do with being reframed — after all, if we get stabbed, we don't blame the wound for bleeding. I believe that dreams are an important tool in this realisation, that if we listen to them, really listen to them, they will help us to listen to ourselves.

Dreams often influence how I work. If I'm quite taken with a subject — which happens often — it can and will infiltrate my dreams. I can wake up with a paragraph or just a phrase already written, as with some of this book. This has happened since I was 15, when once I woke in the night and started to scribble all sorts of words on the walls next to my bed. The words became a small collection of poetry, and a rush of creativity followed. I feel like that night was the first step on the way to becoming an author.

I've been actively engaging with my dreams and visions a lot more over the last decade. It wasn't something I just woke up and did as a practice. It slowly happened, and I had to make a conscious effort for it to happen — in fact, I had to take herbs to enhance the actions, and I experimented with some mugwort. I was at a loose end one evening, as the kids were asleep and Emma was on the phone to her sister. I fancied a drink or two. It had been a few years since I'd written my third book, *Brewing Britain*, and the amount of beer I kept in the house had dwindled to almost nothing. I then found a couple of old bottles of mugwort IPA.

Mugwort, *Artemisia vulgaris*, is well known as a herb that helps to induce lucid dreaming.[19,20] It has been used in many cultures across the world.[21] Despite this widespread usage, scientific studies are rather hard to come by;[22] I mean, it is on the edge of woo-woo, after all. Still, there is some evidence to back up the claims, albeit anecdotal. For example, one YouTuber suggests that mugwort acts as a 'pathway to lucid dreaming';[23] another suggests that her dreams act as a 'healing experience',[24] and one guy states that 'last night feels like a whole week ago ... I remember all of them [his dreams]'.[25]

As with anything to do with our dreams, theories of divinatory dreaming never seem too far away. We've been interpreting dreams in this way for a long time. In Western tradition, at least, the Bible story of Joseph might be the most famous example.

> *Then Pharaoh said to Joseph, 'In my dream I was standing on the bank of the Nile, when out of the river there came up seven cows, fat and sleek, and they grazed among the reeds. After them, seven other cows came up — scrawny and very ugly and lean. I had never seen such ugly cows in all the land of Egypt. The lean, ugly cows ate up the seven fat cows that came up first. But even after they ate them, no one could tell that they had done so; they looked just as ugly as before. Then I woke up.*
>
> *'In my dream I saw seven heads of grain, full and good, growing on a single stalk. After them, seven other heads sprouted — withered and thin and scorched by the east wind. The thin heads of grain swallowed up the seven good heads. I told this to the magicians, but none of them could explain it to me.'*
>
> *Then Joseph said to Pharaoh, 'The dreams of Pharaoh are one and the same. God has revealed to Pharaoh what he is about to do. The seven good cows are seven years, and the seven good heads of grain are seven years; it is one and the same dream. The seven lean, ugly cows that came up afterward are seven years, and so are the seven worthless heads of grain scorched by the east wind: They are seven years of famine.'*[26]

The king then stores a load of food from the seven good years and feeds his people during the seven bad. Bingo bango, the King's dream saves everyone from famine, and they are all happy. No one knows if this is true. That's immaterial, really; I find that religious texts are often about finding wisdom relevant to yourself and your personal situation. That lots of religions remain relevant because this wisdom helps people. What this bit of text does do, however, is help to perpetuate the idea that dreams can be prophetic.

With this sort of cultural heritage behind me, it was no wonder, then, that when I experienced a really vivid mugwort IPA dream, I was taken by the idea that it was a prophetic dream. Unlike the king in the Joseph story, this belief had disastrous financial consequences for me.

When I opened my mugwort IPA, I not only told myself that I'd remember my dreams, I held on to this belief that they might be divinatory. Long before AI had become as ubiquitous as it is now, I dreamed of a world where artificially intelligent cars and mobile phones were one entity, and that they'd started to inject themselves into the young, turning them into their slaves. These entities were programmed with a bloodlust. The dream was so vivid that I took 18 months out of my writing and foraging work to study scriptwriting. It felt like an important piece of work, like something I had to warn the world about.

The thing is, when you start using credit cards to pay yourself, you have to be pretty sure of yourself and that your chosen path will eventually pay off — I read something that suggested scriptwriters take around ten years to get noticed. This was too long; I was already toying with the idea of filing for bankruptcy. The script still lies on an old hard drive, unfinished — I came to my senses and put my mind back to actually earning money. So if intelligent cars do take over the world, I humbly apologise for not doing enough about it when I could.

The next time I really experimented with mugwort was slightly more controlled. One summer's night, after a particularly exhausting emotional time, I decided I wanted to lose myself in a dream. I made myself a mugwort tea by adding a generous pinch (two teaspoons) of dried mugwort to some hot water and infusing it for ten mintes.

Mugwort, I've found, can vary greatly in strength from place to place, year to year. Often, I think, you can smell how good it will be. There is a scent — I think it is the chemical thujone — which is common to mugwort, wormword, tansy and, to a lesser extent, yarrow. A sort of herbal scent, akin to the one you might pick out of a drink of green chartreuse, a smell that reminds many people of childhoods spent by a river — the smell of tansy being brushed past. You might also mistake it for cannabis. I could smell that this particular batch was rather strong.

I didn't need much.

Shortly after drinking the tea, I went to bed, sleeping soundly at first. Then fitfully; my dreams were vivid and plentiful, and they helped. I'd been having trouble connecting to a friend. Well, to be frank, he'd been nothing short of a massive pain in the arse. I was not getting work at the time (which he knew) and he was getting loads — a fact that he kept on reminding me of. I dreamed that he was a turtle in a pond full of murky water — lost and helpless. The dream helped me realised that his showing off was a defence mechanism, that he felt my jealousy of him opening a gulf between us and didn't know what to do. I cleared the water in the dream and then did the same in real life — having a frank discussion about how I really felt. Instead of being jealous and defensive, we managed to share how we felt. The symbolism in dreams can be highly personal. I don't believe that dream dictionaries tell us anything that could be as useful as the study of your own dreams, along with your own intuition.

The morning after the dream, I picked up a tiny book called *A Medieval Herbal* by Jenny De Gex. It described mugwort as a plant used to treat anxiety. It had worked for me; it had given me an insight into my own anxiety.

Anxiety is repeating brain patterns. To overcome anxiety, we have to find a way to disrupt these. This is why meditation or fly agaric mushrooms work. I realised that mugwort, at least on me, acted like a very mild version of a trip or an evening of meditation. I didn't realise then how useful the experience had been. It offered me a different way of seeing a problem; it helped me to find my own influence in a situation.

That mugwort experience helped to unlock something. It helped me to rise above the noise of a problem; often the stress and immediacy of a problem can cloud our judgement. Sometimes it is only distance that gives us the answer; problems are rarely solved in the heat of the moment, after all. My dreaming was becoming that distance; I'd find insights to help me in daily life. I don't drink mugwort to access any more. I'm not entirely sure that it's good for you due to the levels of thujone, and I really would not recommend it becoming habitual.

The active ingredient in mugwort is thujone, and I spoke

to Khaled M. Abass, PhD, a European registered toxicologist from the Research Unit of Biomedicine at the University of Oulu, Finland, about it. He told me that the 'Committee of Herbal Medicinal Products gives two different maximum daily intakes, 3 and 5 mg of thujone/person (70 kg). However, Occurrences of alpha- and beta-thujone in plants depend on plants, batch, seasons, and origins.' In other words, plants have different levels of thujone depending on where they are.

Animal studies, which sometimes feel like an open door to psychopathic behaviour, don't help that much, either. One gave stupidly high thujone concentrations to animals,[27] and within a few minutes almost all of them died. Another,[28] led by an only slightly less psychopathic scientist, gave four groups of 10 female and 10 male rats various doses (0 mg, 5 mg, 10 mg and 20 mg) of thujone (per kilogram of weight), six times a week for 14 weeks. There was no observable effect reported in the 10 mg doses for males and 5 mg for females. At the highest doses, there were convulsions in nine females and six males, while in the 10 mg group only one female convulsed, and this was on Day 38. Further, there were three deaths in the female rats and one male death. The take-home from these studies is the same with any drug — or activity, for that matter — moderation is the key.

Moderation is indeed the key in how you react to your own dreams. Moderation and a little reflection. As I write, I feel like I've had a little revelation about my dream of bloodthirsty AI cars. What I now think my dream was trying to tell me was that I was getting a feeling of being left behind, of being out of touch with the world. I was trying to publish a book about wild cocktails at the time, my then agent was ill, and no one from the literary agency thought it a good idea to pick up her slack. My emails had remained unanswered for over a year — all other work had dried up, too. My beer book hadn't sold as I'd expected, and I was living in a new area with few friends to hand. I was also a new dad and was feeling quite anxious about doing the right thing. In short, I was lonely and felt like a failure.

Had I reflected on the dream, and seen that I was spending too much time on social media comparing myself to others, I might have seen this link with the 'killer technology'. The main protagonist in the dream was isolated from her own family; perhaps I could have opened up to my partner. She was also isolated from her wider community — maybe I should have simply left the house. Instead, I took it to mean I should try a total career shift into a genre that is notoriously difficult to penetrate and, even when you do, is rather precarious — not the best move. I also isolated myself further by obsessing with the notion that I needed to change *the world* rather than just my own world, and sat and wrote alone. Still, I'm not about to beat myself up about it; wisdom is, after all, always so easy with hindsight.

Dreams and visions can be powerful influences. It's easy to dismiss them, as the leading hypothesis about the function of dreams does, attributing their existence to the rather bland idea that they only aid memory retrieval.[29] In my experience, dreams can help to balance us, they can give direction and meaning, they can help in everyday situations. Next time someone suggests you follow your dream, perhaps sit back and work out what your dream was trying to tell you first. And, once again, I really do apologise about our AI mobile phone/car hybrid overlords.

NEW WILD YOUR NIGHT-TIME

Try to build up to spending at least five hours a day outdoors. You can do this by taking breaks outside. If you have a garden, consider creating a space where you can work outside. Walk to nearby shops instead of driving.

Turn off all electronic items at night-time, and switch off your phone at least three hours before you sleep.

Keep a dream diary next to your bed. If you sleep next to someone, find a compromise for how you might work this without disturbing them too much. Take your time studying your own dreams and be mindful of how the symbolism pertains to your own life.

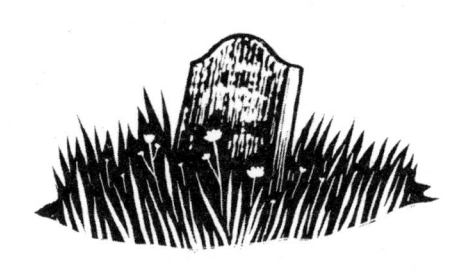

CHAPTER EIGHT

Death

'Death smiles at us all, all a man can do is smile back.'
MARCUS AURELIUS

Two days ago, I walked my familiarly wild route, the route I take when I need a slice of the natural world without having to travel. It's 1,000 steps from where I sit typing this, and it leads me through the natural burial ground at the local cemetery, Arnos Vale. They've been burying people in shallower graves, without traditional coffins, and dressed in all-natural fibres here for the last five years. The burials are sporadic; there is no real pattern to them — you might get two in a month then nothing for the next four. October is at an end; the worm casts are up, forming tiny little mounds around the earth trodden bare by dog walkers. The place is lighter than it used to be, more open due to ash dieback. Piles of ash logs are mounting up; the chainsaws have been busy this year as the cull continues. There is enough surviving ash to carpet the floor with its leaves, some of the first in the forest to drop.

The sight of these cuts sometimes upsets me; I feel a grief when I find areas of dappled shade gone in an afternoon, the character of the forest-cum-cemetery changing overnight. It's become a fact of life, and I'm forced to bear it. The cemetery is, after all, one of Bristol's most visited 'attractions'. Diseased trees that shed heavy branches randomly might be good for business in one way, but ultimately, having someone die in your cemetery makes it a net negative effective. But the forest recovers; life goes on and returns in abundance. There are more rats, and they are fatter; they join the squirrels for the acorn harvest; the oak trees now have a bigger area to spread into and flourish. Grasses and opportunistic second batches of nettles are fed by the decaying bodies of this year's dead. Wildflowers such as rosebay willowherb and lady's bedstraw are now becoming widespread; they, too, have new territory that once wasn't there. Death leads to an inevitable change, and I might as well accept it, especially when it looks this good.

This place is as familiar as my own home; I visit most days. I know the smells, I know if someone is approaching and often where from, and I know which birds I expect to hear, which animals make it their home. Mostly, I know what to expect from the place. But one morning, as I approached the burial site, something stopped me in my tracks. I felt like I might be intruding on something, the feeling pushing me back, telling me to use caution. I didn't feel in danger; I just knew I needed to be respectful. This had happened before, a couple of times. The first when I visited Edinburgh, not long after my mother-in-law died. I felt her close family needed their space. The second was from a much more ancient time — well, sort of.

I'd taken Khloe to the Bristol Museum and Art Gallery to see the touring VR exhibition of the ancient cave art at Lascaux. She'd been before and loved it. I was keen to *explore* the caves myself. I put on the visor, and I was there in the cave, ensconced in its narrow passages. Suddenly, I was in a place devoid of the artificial distractions of city life — it was great. But something didn't feel right; there was that sense of intrusion. It felt like I shouldn't be there, like I was being pushed back, like this place was personal and sacred. I took off the visor and pondered for a second, rationalising what I was feeling. I look over at Khloe; she was already kneeling up and moving about the caves. I decided that it was OK to continue — I mean, I had paid £11 for the experience, after all! I concluded that the damage had been done; if this place was sacred, then someone else had broken that by filming it. That moment made me question the ethics of digging up bones and disturbing the ancient burial sites of our ancestors — was it right to do so just so that people like me could use the findings as a footnote in a book? I always felt uneasy when I saw bones on show at museums, or documentaries where archaeologists hold up skulls. I could imagine how I'd feel if someone found Emma's bones in the future, or my kids', and then paraded them around or put them in a glass case for everyone to gawp at. I doubted I'd like it very much.

The caves felt like they might be a holy place. I pondered whether the animal paintings were actually depictions of something akin to the spirit animals of departed friends and relatives. Whether the blurred lines between the dream world, imagination, and the spirit realm all joined together in those caves. I wondered how the images would look when flickering in firelight or to someone who had taken mushrooms. I wondered, most of all, what drumming might sound like in there, if it echoed around and gave those who stood inside a link with those they were grieving. The dead might not be buried here, but this might be a site of ancient grief. A place to honour the dead. I've started to question whether whatever had happened in those caves was powerful enough to be felt thousands of years later.

The same feeling of intruding on grief at the cemetery felt fresher — if picking up on grief can feel fresh! So much so that I looked to see if there were any mourners around; I felt sure there would be. When I had felt pushed away in Edinburgh, it had been due to being close to very raw grief.

I cross paths with mourners at the same spot in the cemetery about once a month; as the site fills up, more have appeared. Luckily, there is a side path that means I can leave them in peace; they are often so consumed in their own grief that I can skirt around them unnoticed. But I didn't have to do that on this particular day; no one was about. So what was going on? Quite by chance, I found out later that day that three people I know, one of whom is one of my closest friends, were there grieving. Over a pint, my friend confided in me, telling me how he thought his two daughters were coping well with the loss of their mum. But the huge outpouring of grief at the gravesite had told him different. Had I really felt the essense of grief, or was something else going on? Had I simply expected to feel grief in a graveyard, had I noticed extra flowers over some of the graves? Had there been little cues that reminded me of my need to stay alert, ready for a quick, respectful detour? Or had something happened that seems impossible to our minds — had I picked up on some kind of emotional residue?

When I ponder things such as this, I'm reminded that scientific thought and ideas are always changing, that an open mind in journalism, science, music, and anything that is shared with the public is the sharpest tool in our box. I think of all the ideas that have been overturned: Flat Earth, clear-cutting of forests, and *axis mundi*.[1] *Axis mundi* was/is the cross-cultural belief that the Earth was/is at the centre of the universe, an idea that was overturned when Nicolaus Copernicus and Galileo looked out and saw that the Earth moves around the sun. But the instruments to measure emotional residue don't exist — will the technology ever, and *can* it ever, exist? I also understand that my tactics in trying to convince you of it sound like textbook evasion techniques.[2]

This really is third-rail science;* there is no way the scientific community wants to tackle a subject that is seemingly so out there — it's not as if we are a spiritual society in search of such things. The single person I could find studying this area was Krishna Savani.[3] He firstly asked participants in a study if emotions could travel outside the body. The First Nation Americans he asked thought they could, while most of the other participants — Americans with Western ideology — said they couldn't, illustrating an obvious difference in cultural beliefs. Then he put notices on two doors; one said that someone had been sitting there

---

* The third rail is the electrified rail on the Underground. Touch it, and you die. Anything considered to be 'third rail' is so toxic that touching it might end your career.

recalling happy events; the other said someone had sat there recalling unhappy events. He told his interviewees to pick a room to fill in their questionnaires. The majority picked the 'happy' room,[4] and he concluded that at some level many of us believe in emotional residue. The fact that this phenomenon exists, however, still remains unmeasured and answered.

As does the idea of life after death — science still struggles to understand why a belief in the afterlife still exists.[5] Many humans find it hard to imagine that we don't just go on, and so life after death is an *ipso facto* belief. We think, therefore we live on. Still, there are others who simply refuse to believe there is anything but this life, most famously Richard Dawkins,[6] who seems to revel in the fact that there is 'nothing else'. He jokes that the afterlife would be, 'incredibly tedious after the first 1,000 years'.[7] Are science and the afterlife really that incompatible?

Francis Crick thought so. He was a fellow Northamptonian (born yards away from my upper school), and one of the people who pulled a fast one on Rosalind Franklin to take all the glory for laying the groundwork for the structure of DNA.[8] He helped to popularise the theory of 'nothing else' in modern culture. In his 1994 book, *The Astonishing Hypothesis*, he suggests that we are nothing more than DNA. 'Your sense of personal identity and free will, are in fact no more than the behaviour of a vast assembly of nerve cells and their associated molecules.'[9]

Thankfully, when the chips are down, most of us do believe in a life after death. In a famous 2002 study, American scientist Jesse Bering asked students a series of questions beginning with thoughts about an afterlife in which most students suggested that they did indeed believe.[10] However, many students ticked a box that stated 'What we think of as the "soul," or conscious personality of a person, ceases permanently when the body dies'. These students were dubbed 'extinctivists'.

The students were then given a short fictitious paragraph to read:

> *RICHARD WAVERLY was a 37-year-old history teacher. One day he was driving to work, tired after a late night and hungry from skipping breakfast. He was also in a bad mood following a row with his wife, who he suspected of having an affair. At a busy junction, he lost control, drove into a telegraph pole and was thrown through the windscreen. The paramedics said he was dead before he hit the pavement.*

In order to find out what the students really thought, Bering continued with a series of further questions including, 'Do you think Richard knows he is dead?' and, 'Do you think he wishes he had told his wife he loved her before he died?' They were somewhat trick questions, designed to catch the students out. If Richard knows he's dead, then there is continued mental cognition even after death; moreover, if he wishes he'd told his wife, then his emotions continue. Of course, as you'd expect, those who believed in an afterlife attributed continued mental cognition to Richard. But, more remarkably, 32 per cent of the extinctivists thought that emotional states can continue after death. A further 36 per cent also thought that Richard, despite being dead and ceasing to have a personality, did indeed know he was dead. Meaning all but one third of the small group of exinctivist students actually believed there was something else.

I'm not sure if I've ever believed in the unimaginative *nothing else* view of the afterlife. The view seems cold and inhuman to me. It also feels like a cultural hindrance; Dawkins might be comfortable with the idea, and my friend Marric, too, but most of us don't want to believe that this life is all there is — it's quite terrifying. This means death has become a highly taboo subject in our culture. We might have rituals that deal with the body, but it feels like we are losing some of the rituals that help the bereaved emotionally, that help with our own souls. I believe that this is where our secular ideology fails us greatly. We may not live in the centre of the universe, but we still live in the centre of our own personal universe — the universe of our own experiences, the world of the countless cells, microbiota, and fungi that make us up. Take away a belief in the afterlife and reduce the rituals around death, and we are left with cold comfort.

I spoke about death to a friend in the Outdoor Writer's and Photographers guild, the other day, about my own death. 'It's refreshing to hear someone talk about death,' she said, adding, 'People don't — they don't even like the word "death".' It's not a subject I shy away from; one of the reasons, perhaps, that I'm not always invited back to social events. I walk through the cemetery almost daily and read the language on graves dating back over the last 200 years. I see hints of the stories they tell: young lovers who died within months of each other, mothers who buried more than one of their offspring. It's a place where people are resting, or have passed on — there are euphemisms everywhere, and rarely any mention of the words 'death' or 'dying'. Is this because what happens next remains a mystery to modern science and the cultural view of millions of Westerners?[11]

Perhaps this view sums up our culture more than any other. We hate death and prolong the dying process. Hospitals will spend one third of their budgets on people in the last three years of life.[12] Our attitudes influence the clinical way we treat the corpse; the majority of Americans,[13] Australians, and British people choose to cremate their dead.[14] It's far easier and more clinical that way — who wants to deal with a body when you can deal with a box full of ashes instead?

Compare this to the Toraja, mountain people from Sulawesi, Indonesia, who, as part of their funeral rites, will exhume the bodies of their dead and change their clothes long after they they have passed. Here, they treat death and grieving as a social gathering. The knotty and messy emotions of grieving take time to work their way through us; it's also a slow process, and so, in this culture, are the rituals around it. The bodies of the dead can be preserved and then kept in a house until such a time as the family can afford the funeral.[15] The Toraja believe, as do I, that the spirit will live for a while in this world until it begins its journey to the next realm.

I felt this need for a better grieving process most acutely after a friend I'd known since school jumped in front of a train. He'd been given one of the 19 million prescriptions written for GlaxoSmithKline's antidepressant drug Seroxat — the drug that was linked to an increase in the risk of suicide in some patients after it had been cleared for use in a flawed 2001 study.[16,17] I'd not long been offered a six-figure publishing deal when it happened, a great career leap from the low-paid and menial temp jobs I was working at that point.

My grieving was helped by organising his funeral. I was one of the pall bearers; I carried the coffin and helped to lower it into the ground. These, it could be argued were distracting techniques. They kept me away from having to face up to my emotions. Like many men, I was being an action-focused griever.[18] I always like to be busy at a time of death. Stopping and doing nothing becomes a messy process, and after my friend died, I didn't want it to get in the way of what was — and is — my dream job. For a while I thought I'd mastered it, scheduling time to grieve.[19] A month ought to do it, I thought. I sat and thought about him; I had a grieving spot — a chair in my living room — and I curled myself up in it for two hours a day, every day. It sort of worked; it allowed me to get on and finish the book. But it sort of didn't, too; I drank a lot, I carried it around. If you read the dreams chapter, I wonder if all I did was lock it away.

Grief might stalk us all — that's a cheery thought — but there is much debate as to whether or not we are the only species which is aware of the inevitability of death.[20] Many species grieve: dogs, chimpanzees, and elephants, for example.

Victoria was a Kenyan elephant who died in June 2013. For three weeks after her death, her body became a source of interest to both her relatives and unrelated elephants as they came to visit, her own son and daughter being the most visceral in their response. Her daughter showed visible signs of distress, while the son was more tactile in his response, and kept trying to push her body over.

We may not, and we may never, fully understand the grieving process of elephants. I often think I don't understand my own — it's different every time, after all. Suicides are always hard; I've been losing friends that way since I was a teenager and, if anything, it gets harder. Yet some deaths — my nan, for instance — have felt easier to deal with, I think for many reasons. She was old, in her eighties; she'd been ill already; and, most importantly, I got a chance to say goodbye.

Just before her last stroke, my parents took the four of us out for a pub lunch for Nan's birthday. Nan sat opposite me and just held my hands and looked into my eyes, ignoring my parents whom she saw all the time. We talked, and she insisted on doing this for the whole two hours we were out. It felt awkward at first, and my mum was a little twitchy. Don't forget we are British, after all — anyone who has ridden the Tube will know that public emotions are not our thing! But then I relaxed into the moment, enjoying it for what it was. I now feel she was saying goodbye. When her death came, it just felt like the next step for her, and the grief didn't feel so painful. She'd gone, and I could accept that. I hope I get a chance to do the same for my children, and grandchildren if I have any.

Perhaps it was that closeness at the pub that made the grief easier; it felt like she'd prepared me, that she had decreed it should be easier for me. Maybe she'd known she was about to go. For some, those words will rest heavily on the page. There are two things wrong with that statement, after all. Firstly, it assumes some kind of prediction, and that's pseudoscience; secondly, as I've mentioned, we simply don't want to accept the fact that one day we will die. How, then, could someone both readily accept their own death and predict when it was going to happen?

An experiment published in *NeuroImage* certainly fuels the debate;[21] it concludes that we naturally shield ourselves from existential threats by shutting down our sense of self when we think about death. We file it away; it's something that happens to others and not to ourselves. This, it is argued, is our defence mechanism in a death-phobic world. But are we really shutting down a part of our brain for this reason? I wonder if that response highlights the idea that science reflects how society currently thinks about something.

We might instead consider that the brain is actually rewiring itself to a life without the person we greive for in it. All the predictions we once had for our life will have changed. This is what grief researcher Mary-Frances O'Connor suggests.[22] We feel this not only in our minds but in our bodies, too: blood pressure can rise, bringing along with it a host of associated health problems. It's important, then, to ensure that as we rewire, we do so in a nurturing environment. Nature will help, and so will being around caring individuals. This is something that religion can bring to the party.

If it is said that many of the world's religions exist only as a way to mitigate this fear of death,[23] then they also help to repair the mind and body after someone dies — something my devoutly Christian nan found. Nan wasn't always religious, no more than anyone of her generation was. She turned to Christianity. Her second-born son, Roy Hamilton, was hit by a car when out on his moped. He was only 17, brain death occurred, and it was Nan who had to make the decision to turn off the life support. She remained distraught for quite some time afterwards. That was until one night when Roy came to visit. He sat on the edge of her bed and told her he was doing okay where he was. For my nan, that was proof enough that there is another life after this, and every Sunday from then onwards, she attended a Christian church service. Often humans will turn to religion at trying times.[24] But religion did more than just mitigate a fear of death for Nan; my granddad had stopped her from leaving the house. It gave her a freedom she got nowhere else; it gave her community and a chance to sing. She *went rogue* on occasion, as my dad might put it, and attended a Baptist church. I went along once, and it was much more fun than our regular church — the singing was certainly much more alive!

To reduce my nan's experience of religion to just a mitigation of the fear of death is to do it a disservice. Whatever it was that she saw or felt that evening, it helped. In the years before her own death, she had a stroke and some health issues. I think she had a good idea of when she might die, and her faith meant she was also ready for it.

I've met people in the same position. The psychiatric hospital where I worked had three wards: a general one, a high-security ward, and one for elderly patients. I've also worked on a couple of cruise ships. In both settings, I met people with not long to live, and many had an acceptance of death. Not everyone — some seemed very bitter about the idea, and some would mention it often, if only to hear some reassurance that they were going to live for longer. But there was certainly a grace and serenity about those who felt it coming and accepted their fate. People who had fulfilled their final wishes in coming on the cruise would declare that they could 'die now'. I spoke at length to one ship's vicar about this and many other religious matters; as both a retired nurse and a vicar, she'd seen a lot of death. She stated that not only had she developed a sense of when people were going to die, but she thought that many people chose to die — letting go. Of course, this is something that older people understandably find easier. The younger we are, the more likely we are to feel cheated by our allocated time.[25]

I've not been around at the end of anyone's life; the closest relatable experience is being present for an animal's death. Before Emma and I decided to have children, we thought we'd do a practice run and keep a pet. We decided on two gerbils and, being unrelated, we painstakingly introduced them to each other. Eventually, they got along fine and would cuddle up as they slept. It was impossibly cute, and we felt like we were parenting. Great, you might think, until you remind yourself of the subject of this chapter.

To cut a long story short, one morning I found one of the gerbils dying — attacked by his gerbil housemate and in a very sorry state. He'd normally run a mile when we tried to scoop him up, but that morning he didn't fight at all as I gently put him into my hand. I sat back on the sofa, holding his delicate, battered body in my palm. I watched his laboured breathing. There was something of the infinite about it, an echo in the air. Time stands still when death is out stalking.

I looked down at him and felt something leave his body as he breathed his last breath, leaving the shell of his existence behind. I felt the same thing — his *spirit*? — when we buried him; it was if he was off saying goodbye. His housemate died shortly after, and we never got another pet. In fact, we left it a little while until we did eventually have children — about another six or seven years. The experience might not have prepared me for parenthood, but it did help me with a period of time when we seemed to experience a number of deaths that all followed our gerbils'.

Whatever you want to call the feeling of our gerbil being present after death — the soul, a ghost, his spirit, a useful hallucination — it wasn't anything new to me. I've felt like I've experienced the presence of many people after their death. It started with Doug, my childhood friend who died when I was 17 (see Chapter Two). Sitting in a caravan where he had spent a summer, both a close friend, Jass, and I noticed him. If you have ever felt like you know who's entered a room even when you have your back to them, it's that feeling. We stayed for a week, and once we noticed his presence, it felt like he was there, with us, constantly — in fact, he wouldn't go away. Over the course of our holiday, we met two local girls, got on very well, and then invited them both back to the caravan. Doug stayed around even when we wanted to be alone. We agreed that it became a little uncomfortable at these times. I don't know if Jass was humouring me, but I do know that it brought me some comfort and, either way, I was glad that Jass agreed.

I felt my gran's presence when we first moved into this house — her legacy afforded us the down payment. I've also felt many people whom I was close to — a great-aunt, my mother-in-law — and some that I wasn't so close to — an old boss whom I only met a handful of times, and my friend's wife, a woman to whom I'd said fewer than three sentences.

More recently, I started to feel the presence of freshly interred bodies in the newly established natural burial site at the local cemetery — people I've never met. It's a place that is almost like another character in this book, the place where I get a slice of nature and from where I ate something wild every day for year.

It's a place I have a deep affinity with; the act of eating something from there daily made it feel like this area in which people are now buried is part of me. In a very real sense, it is: the nutrients in plants I ate from that area made up my bones, hair, vital organs, the eyes I see through, and the brain I think with.

It is a special place for those interred there, too. They become anonymous: there, no one is looking at the dates or names on their gravestones for some history project, no would-be parents are looking for baby names, no one is taking the piss out of their name, no writers are looking for inspiration for stories. Those buried there simply become part of the world again from whence they came.

People leave rocks and flowers, free of plastic, poking out of the mounds — a couple I've noticed now have wooden crosses on them, which will rot. It means that, once buried, your footprint is a mound of earth, which in time becomes indistinguishable from the rest of the forest. In the few years that the site has been operational, some graves have already almost vanished. Flushes of nettles feed merrily on the new abundance of nutrients in the soil. Enchanter's nightshade sways magically and gently in the dappled light. Trees are starting to take root: hazel, sycamore, ash (although doomed by dieback), hornbeam, and oak. It's a beautiful place, made more so by allowing this process. You may think that this adds poignancy to the place, and for some it does. Personally, I feel it adds serenity and hope — it's all part of the 3.5-billion-year cycle of life.

Of these graves, two stand out, two I've had funny feelings around. I've walked across that site for many years, since long before it became a natural burial area. I didn't know the bodies had started going in and one day, as I approached, I felt cold all over — a feeling of death (funnily enough) befell me, and it sent a chill down my spine. My mind's eye showed a morgue. A few months later, I felt something very different. I was near a grave and I started to giggle; I couldn't help myself. It was the strangest feeling and, once it had started, it didn't stop. For the next six months or more, all I could do was giggle as I walked near.

I'm not certain why I feel this — do I really sense the dead? Perhaps it's a symptom of undiagnosed bipolar condition; I do, after all, have quite profound ups and downs.[26] This would certainly make sense of some of the other visions and hallucinations that I experience. Perhaps I'm deluded, or perhaps the effects of taking LSD from the age of 14 have made their mark. I can find a host of reasons that would dismiss these occurrences, reasons that could easily be squared with rational science — all reasons I'd cite when discussing it with someone who might refuse to believe in something spiritual, especially if I was feeling like it might hamper the conversation and therefore the joy of someone's company. But the truth is, none of these explanations sit comfortably. The idea that I feel the dead, conversely, does.

The one thing that each of these manifestations, hallucinations or whatever they are have in common is that (with the exception of my mother-in-law) by the time I felt the dead person's presence, I was not in the throes of grief. They came at a moment of calm, when my mind was relaxed. I thought little about this until I read *The Madness of Grief* by Richard Coles. In the preface he speaks about Mary Magdalene's grief on finding Jesus' tomb empty, as depicted in Titian's *Noli me Tangere*, which hangs in the National Gallery in London. Jesus apparently said to her, 'Do not touch me,' which seems a little harsh — but, as Richard explains, though many assume that Jesus was rejecting her, was he predicting her reaction to his death? The translation from the Latin to the traditional Greek Orthodox reads a little differently:

> *Do not cling to me, for I have not yet ascended to the Father; but go to my brothers and say to them, 'I am ascending to My Father and your Father, to My God and your God.'* (John 20:17)

Upon reading that, I felt I understood something of my grieving process. Grief can feel like walking with wet shoes through a bog with the sleet hammering against your face. Every emotion, every fibre in your body is set on getting through that moment; at times it feels like there is little room for much else. Sleep can be the only escape, and instead of waking up from a nightmare, you awake into one. Yet, the clouds do eventually clear, the bog gives way to firm ground. The feelings lessen in intensity as time passes. Ebbing and flowing throughout the process, one day you are fine and the next you are bogged down again. Through the cycles of grief, the times when you stop clinging to the life of the dead person become more frequent, when the enormity of the emotion rests for a while; this is when acceptance starts to take the stage. It is during these moments, for me, that I feel most likely to sense the presence of the dead. And when you are not clinging to the idea that the person is still here in an earthly form, it helps to shorten the grieving period.

When I speak to others about sensing their loved ones, it can be a comfort to them. It helps to think that something of that person is still around — maybe that's all these feelings are for. To offer some relief. I wonder, too, if 17,000 years ago in a cave in France, a fistful of mushrooms and the beat of a drum and the flicker of firelight gave comfort to those who had lost loved ones, too. In fact, I think I might start looking for a cave now, somewhere with great resonance. Somewhere that might help people to grieve me after my death.

NEW WILD YOUR GRIEVING PROCESS

The grieving process is unique and can be one of the most difficult aspects of our lives to come to terms with. Don't be in a rush to get on with your life; allow yourself time.

To help others, give them the space to grieve and permission to feel whatever emotion seems right.

Learn to listen.

Suggest walks or time outdoors, and just be there for one another.

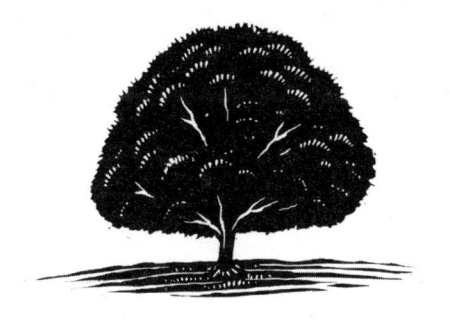

Further Reading

The books below surround me right now, on the shelves that circle my writing desk. Some have been with me for many years; some are recent additions to my library. All have inspired or informed me in some way or other, and I hope these great minds inspire you, too.

Chapter One: Life

Anderson, M. Kat. *Tending the Wild: Native American Knowledge and the Management of California's Natural Resources.* University of California Press, 2013.

Gunn, Emma. *Never Mind the Burdocks: a year of foraging in the British Isles.* Emma Gunn, 2014.

Hamilton, Andy. *Booze for Free.* Eden Project Books, 2017.

— *The First-Time Forager: a complete beginner's guide to Britain's edible plants* (National Trust). HarperCollins, 2024.

Irving, Miles. *The Forager Handbook: a guide to the edible plants of Britain*. Ebury, 2009.
Lambert, Rachel. *Seaweed Foraging in Cornwall and the Isles of Scilly*. Alison Hodge, 2016.
Lewis-Stempel, John. *The Wild Life: a year of living on wild food*. Black Swan, 2016.
Masters, Susanne. *Wild Waters*. Vertebrate Publishing, 2021.
Nozedar, Adele. *The Garden Forager*. Random House, 2015.
Rensten, John. *The Edible City*. Pan Macmillan, 2016.
Thayer, Samuel. *The Forager's Harvest: a guide to identifying, harvesting, and preparing edible wild plants*. Forager's Harvest, 2006.
Wilde, Mo. *The Wilderness Cure*. Simon & Schuster, 2023.
Wright, John. *The Forager's Calendar*. Profile Books, 2019.

Chapter Two: Consciousness

Allegro, John. *The Sacred Mushroom and the Cross*. Hodder & Stoughton, 1970.
Devereux, Paul. *The Long Trip*. Penguin, 1997.
Emily Wanderer Cohen. *From Generation to Generation*. Morgan James Publishing, 2018.
Feeney, Kevin M. *Fly Agaric: a compendium of history, pharmacology, mythology & exploration*. Fly Agaric Press, 2020.
Gillett, Ed. *Party Lines*. Pan Macmillan, 2023.
McKenna, Terence. *Food of the Gods: The Search for the Original Tree of Knowledge: a radical history of plants, drugs and human evolution*. Rider, 1999.
Masha, Baba. *Microdosing with Amanita Muscaria*. Simon & Schuster, 2022.
Richard Evans Schultes, et al. *Plants of the Gods: their sacred, healing, and hallucinogenic powers*. Healing Arts Press, 2001.
Shaw, Martin. *Smoke Hole: looking to the wild in the time of the spyglass*.

Chelsea Green Publishing, 2021.
— *Wolf Milk: chthonic memory in the deep wild*. Cista Mystica Press, 2019.
Stamets, Paul. *Psilocybin Mushrooms of the World: an identification guide*. Ten Speed Press, 1996.

Chapter Three: Shelter

Barnhouse, Rebecca. *The Old English Hexateuch*. Medieval Institute Publications, 2000.
Bowman, Katy. *Rethink Your Position*. Propriometrics Press, 2022.
Buzzell, Linda, and Craig Chalquist. *Ecotherapy*. Counterpoint, 2009.
Ivens, Sarah. *Forest Therapy*. Da Capo Lifelong Books, 2018.
Le Corre, Erwan. *The Practice of Natural Movement: reclaim power, health, and freedom*. Victory Belt Publishing Inc., 2019.
Li, Qing. *Forest Bathing: how trees can help you find health and happiness*. Viking, 2018.
Mitchell, Emma. *The Wild Remedy: how nature mends us – a diary*. Michael O'Mara Books Ltd, 2019.
Rybczynski, Witold. *How Architecture Works*. Farrar, Straus and Giroux, 2013.
Shaw, Martin. *Courting the Wild Twin*. Chelsea Green Publishing, 2020.
— *Smoke Hole: looking to the wild in the time of the spyglass*. Chelsea Green Publishing, 2021.
Smyth, Richard. *A Sweet, Wild Note*. Elliott & Thompson, 2018.
Stuart-Smith, Sue. *The Well Gardened Mind: rediscovering nature in the modern world*. William Collins, 2021.

Chapter Four: Bodies

Davies, Patrick, *Where Skylarks Sing*. Caravan Books, 2023.
Enders, Giulia. *Gut: the inside story of our body's most underrated organ*

(revised edition). Greystone Books, 2018.

Finn, Adharanand. *The Rise of the Ultra Runners*. Simon & Schuster, 2019.

Hamblin, James. *Clean*. Penguin, 2020.

Lieberman, Daniel. *Exercised: the science of physical activity, rest and health*. Allen Lane, 2020.

Chapter Five: Music

Chatwin, Bruce. *The Songlines*. Vintage, 1998.

Couzens, Dominic. *A Year of Birdsong*. Batsford Books, 2022.

Devereux, Paul. *Stone Age Soundtracks: the acoustic archaeology of ancient sites*. Vega, 2001.

Diallo, Yaya, and Mitchell Hall. *The Healing Drum: African wisdom teachings*. Destiny Books, 1989.

Drake, Michael. *Shamanic Drumming*. Talking Drum Publications, 2012.

Hollander, Julia. *Why We Sing*. Atlantic Books, 2024.

Levitin, Daniel J. *This Is Your Brain on Music: the science of a human obsession*. Dutton, 2006.

Sacks, Oliver. *Musicophilia*. Picador, 2007.

Chapter Six: Art

Bayne, Tim, et al. *The Oxford Companion to Consciousness*. Oxford University Press, 2014.

Buhner, Stephen Harrod. *Plant Intelligence and the Imaginal Realm*. Simon & Schuster, 2014.

Cameron, Julia. *The Artist's Way Morning Pages Journal: a companion volume to The Artist's Way*. Hay House, 2017.

De Botton, Alain, and John Armstrong. *Art as Therapy*. Phaidon Press Limited, 2013.

Foster, Charles. *Being a Beast*. Profile, 2016

Harvey, Graham. *Animism: respecting the living world*. Hurst & Company, 2017.

Henri, Robert, and Alfredo Valente. *Robert Henri: Painter-Teacher-Prophet*. Cultural Center in association with Fairleigh Dickinson University, 1969.

Lewis-Williams, David. *The Mind in the Cave*. Thames & Hudson, 2002.

Vonnegut, Kurt, and Dan Wakefield. *If This Isn't Nice, What Is?: Advice to the Young: the graduation speeches*. Seven Stories Press, 2014.

West, Keith R. *How to Draw Plants*. The Herbert Press, 1983.

Chapter Seven: Sleep

Bach, Richard. *Jonathan Livingston Seagull*. Simon & Schuster, 1970.

Carroll, Lewis. *Lewis Carroll's Jabberwocky*. StarWalk Kids Media, 2014.

Francis-Baker, Tiffany. *Dark Skies: a journey into the wild night*. Bloomsbury, 2019.

Gooley, Tristan. *Wild Signs and Star Paths*. Hachette UK, 2018.

Robb, Alice. *Why We Dream: the new science behind dreams and why they matter*. Picador, 2019.

Shelley, Mary Wollstonecraft. *Frankenstein, Or, the Modern Prometheus*. Lackington, Hughes, Harding, Mavor & Jones, 1818.

Walker, Matthew P. *Why We Sleep: unlocking the power of sleep and dreams*. Scribner, 2017.

Chapter Eight: Death

Adichie, Chimamanda Ngozi. *Notes on Grief*. 4th Estate, 2021.

Biers, Trish, and Katie Stringer Clary. The Routledge Handbook of Museums, Heritage, and Death. Taylor & Francis, 2023.

Burnett, Elizabeth-Jane. *Twelve Words for Moss*. Random House, 2023.

Coles, The Reverend Richard. *The Madness of Grief: a memoir of love and loss*. Weidenfeld & Nicolson, 2021.

Doughty, Caitlin. *From Here to Eternity: traveling the world to find the good death*. W. W. Norton & Company, 2017.

Lewis, C.S. *A Grief Observed*. Crossreach Publications, 2016.

O'Connor, Mary-Frances. *The Grieving Brain: the surprising science of how we learn from love and loss*. HarperOne, 2022.

General Further Reading

Boyle, Mark. *The Way Home: tales from a life without technology*. Oneworld Publications, 2019.

Du Cann, Charlotte, et al. *Walking on Lava: selected works for uncivilised times*. Chelsea Green Publishing, 2017.

Jung, Carl. *Psychological Types*. Routledge, 1921.

Kingsnorth, Paul, et al. *Uncivilisation: the dark mountain manifesto*. The Dark Mountain Project, 2019.

Laozi. *Tao Te Ching*. Simon & Brown, 2018.

Monbiot, George. *Feral*. University of Chicago Press, 2014.

Sheldrake, Merlin. *Entangled Life: how fungi make our worlds, change our minds, and shape our futures*. S.L., Random House, 2021.

Spikins, Penelope Ann. *How Compassion Made Us Human*. Pen and Sword, 2015.

Thoreau, Henry David. *Walden*. Vintage, 1854.

Wengrow, David, and David Graeber. *The Dawn of Everything*. Farrar, Straus and Giroux, 2021.

Acknowledgements

First of all, I want to thank you — yes, you — the person holding this book, the person who has shown enough interest in what I have to say to pick up this book and to turn to the acknowledgement pages. Thanks.

Although, if you have flicked to this bit because you are someone who I met along the long path I took when creating this book, then hello! I do hope I have included you below. If not, then think about how the brain works — sometimes words that you use all the time don't come to mind. The names of loved ones are forgotten for an instant, or you might go into a room for something important and have no idea why you are there. That is to say, the fact that I haven't included you just means I've forgotten right now, as I type. I trust you'll understand that and forgive me.

Still, hopefully I have remembered enough of you.

This book would not have existed were it not for two women: my partner, Emma, and my transatlantic yogic agent and friend, Kate Johnson of Wolf Literary Services. Both have been patient and have listened and advised as, from the spore of an idea, *New Wild Order* unfurled into what you have in your hands.

I also want to thank my commissioning editor, Simon Wright at Scribe, for seeing the potential in this book. Along with Kitty Liu at Cornell University Press for believing in an early incarnation, and Mireille Harper for much the same, too — both of you just got it straight away, and that positivity reverberates into the bones of an author. Well, into this one, anyway.

Then there are those who do the hard work, the real graft of book production — the team of people at Scribe that beavered away to get this book to this state. I need therefore to give a huge thank-you to Molly Slight for going beyond what was expected and really pulling my words together. You are simply very good at your job, and it doesn't go unnoticed. To Laura Ali, for majestically taking the reins and picking up where Molly left off.

Thanks, too, to Nicola Garrison for expertly working on the book's marketing and publicity, and Richard Humphreys on sales — both of you helped to get this book into as many hands as possible, and I sincerely thank you for that. A big thank-you to my diligent copy-editor, Eleanor Updegraff, too; I hope the reader will agree that you have ensured that reading this book has been stumble-free.

But I also want to thank the booksellers, the book distributers, the warehouse workers, the person who piloted the ship that this book sailed on. Indeed, everyone who has

ACKNOWLEDGEMENTS

had anything to do with getting this book from where it existed, inside my head, to the hard copy that you are now looking at. It's an odd thought for a boy who dreamed of one day having a book out to now have seven, and each one of you helps in that process.

Along the way there have been many others, too, more directly involved with the text of the book, and others who have been interviewed or have given their time and advice with generosity. Some chapters have ended up on the cutting-room floor, not as a fault of these folks — or the quality of their work in informing those chapters — but just due to the nature of the creative process. It can be a brutal beast, and I'm sorry if you didn't fit for whatever reason.

Yet, with that in mind, I don't want anyone's help to go unrecognised, and therefore I thank some of those people who didn't make the cut — Craig Worrall for our many wondrous chats and, of course, your friendship; Joe Hoare for the sessions of laughter yoga when I really needed it, and for your time; Angie Belcher for chatting to me about stand-up comedy.

But onwards to the people who did inform these pages. I want to thank my kids, Loki and Lark, for just being yourselves. The natural way you both engage with world around you has helped inform much of what I intuited in these pages.

Then to the staff at Bristol Libraries, the unseen people who move books around the south-west of England. But to the seen people in the libraries, too, especially to Jonty Bewley, Joy, and Ollie Betts.

To Dr George Moncrieff for your help in convincing me to stop washing so much, Billy Morgan for helping me to give up furniture, Molly Miranda King for helping me to sing and find inner peace, Sarah Larkham (do you add the Hall these days, too?) for the chats about drumming, and, of course, Michelle Leadbetter for your excellent drumming. Sam Hobson for shamanic and tree talk. But also, Ava Maginnis from the Human Nature Project for gently guiding me into a forest bathing session.

I'd like to thank the Bristol Writing group: Mike Manson, Ray Newman, Corinne Dobinson, David Griffiths, Piers Matter, Liz Kalaugher, Chris Barnard, and Kate Sykes for your advice on my early drafts.

To Mark Williams and Jon M. Erlandson for talking seaweed, and to Jane Carswell, Lynton Davidson, and Sharon McHarrie for inviting me up Islay. To Ru Kenyon, Rob Gould, Alex McAllister-Lunt, Dave Winnard, and Martin Bailey for foraging chat and adventures. Sam Webster and Emma Cronin for your enthusiasm and encouragement for my Substack and the themes that cross-fed this book. Also, of course, to all at the Association of Foragers, my second family. To Rachel Lambert for the seaweed recipe and fun chats.

Thanks for the design work of Derek Edwards and Nick Moyle as I worked my way into figuring out what this book would be. Writing advice from Nathan Filer. The support, photos, and kind ear of my good friend Royston Hunt, who often just guides my thoughts into directions I may have never considered.

To Garth Nuade for chatting about the inner self, even on a day off.

To Sausage John Atkinson for the loan of your woodland, and to Nev Kilkenny for offering, too. To the staff, volunteers, and trustees of Arnos Vale Cemetery, and to Bristol Council's parks department, for my special wild place and a cafe in which to sit, contemplate the world, and trip my bollox off.

Of course, I can't forget to mention the amazing group of folks at Bricks' St Anne's House in Bristol. Especially Lou and Georgia, for helping me to feel welcome and making it easy to be in that group at a time when I needed it.

To Kaye Brennan and Amanda Butler for feeding me when I lived in Nottingham so I could write this, and to Craig Jones, Dave Jennings, Sue Kind, Sam, Luther, Mark, Rod, and Michelle for being mates at that time and being sound folks, too. Sorry I never visited Nottingham again — I will one day!

To Ted Smallbone for driving me and Doug down to Cornwall, and for being a good bloke. To my site party and raving friends: Helen Keen, John Randal, Kelly Wannop, Liz Cooke, Pete Hill, Dean Curtis, Jass Trew, Ashley Potter, Keith Jones, Maria Broome, Neil Steals, Nick Palmer, Scott Pateman, Simon (smit) Smith, Sarah Solley, Nick Dyer, Dave Doyle, Dom Reed-Jones, and Graham Fraiser. Of course, there were more than you guys, but come on, it was 20 years ago and we were all off it (and read the top bit — it doesn't meant I don't care) ... But, go on, better mention Frag Ginbey, Dan Cameron, and Russ Bradshaw, too, even though you never came along.

To the 8th St Albans Cubs and Scout Troop of Northampton circa 1982-1988.

To Richard Jones, Lon Barford, Beccy Golding, Marc Leverton, Nicky Coates, Sol Wilkinson, Johanna Darque, Mark Steeds, and Joe Melia, the folk from my office, for listening to me as I bashed through the very early incarnations of this book.

To Naomi Walmsley for friendship and for chatting to me about your and Dan Westall's experiences living the Stone Age.

To Bruce Parry for giving me a slice of his time, and Miles Irving for helping to put us in touch.

To Nigel Holt, Alison Lee, Lance Workman, and Alison Wadely, the psychology department of Bath Spa University circa 2000-2005. I may have been drunk most of the time, but some of what you taught me did stick after all; it was the spark that made these pages. Alison Lee, suggesting that my voice sang through in my essays was quite influential. And Lance, I think it was you who suggested that depression was an evolutionary overhang — I wasn't having that!

Then I want to thank those who enthusiastically encouraged me as I undertook these challenges. Sophie Bancroft and Skye Lyndsey, you stand out the most in this camp, as do all the staff at Sandy Park Greengrocers, and Jess Clarke and Josephine, too. But also Andy Pole and my Auntie Chris, who deserve a bit of an honorary mention, too. There were more folks than this, but it's late and I want off this computer — but that doesn't mean I don't love you!

To all those wild people, researchers, academics, authors, and filmmakers whose hard work helped to inform these pages. Thanks for offering much of your work as open source. You made this job a lot easier than it was back when I first started it almost a decade ago.

And to my mum and dad for giving me the best start you could in life — the best you could give was always good enough to make me feel loved.

Endnotes

Introduction: The Call of the Wild
1 https://www.spectator.co.uk/article/when-violence-was-the-norm-britain-in-the-1980s/ — retrieved 5/7/2024
2 https://www.stanfordchildrens.org/en/topic/default?id=generalized-anxiety-disorder-gad-in-children-and-teens-90-P02565 — retrieved 13/6/2024
3 Jung, C.G. *Letters Volume 2*. Routledge and Kegan Paul, 1976.
4 https://www.ons.gov.uk/peoplepopulationandcommunity/crimeandjustice/articles/thenatureofviolentcrimeinenglandandwales/yearendingmarch2018 — retrieved 17/7/2024

Chapter One: Life
1 https://www.gov.uk/government/statistics/universal-credit-statistics-29-april-2013-to-12-october-2023/universal-credit-statistics-29-april-2013-to-12-october-2023 — retrieved 6/7/2024
2 https://www.trusselltrust.org/news-and-blog/latest-stats/end-

year-stats/#factsheets — retrieved 6/7/2024
3. https://en.wikipedia.org/wiki/List_of_countries_by_total_wealth — retrieved 6/7/2024
4. Fentahun, M.T. and H. Hager. 'Exploiting locally available resources for food and nutritional security enhancement: wild fruits diversity, potential and state of exploitation in the Amhara region of Ethiopia', *Food Security*, 1, 2009, pp. 207–19.
5. https://www.newscientist.com/article/mg26334980-500-how-ghost-cities-in-the-amazon-are-rewriting-the-story-of-civilisation/ — retrieved 7/7/2024
6. Araújo, R.G., and R.A. Chavez-Santoscoy, R. Parra-Saldívar, E.M. Melchor-Martínez, and H.M. Iqbal. 'Agro-food systems and environment: Sustaining the unsustainable', *Current Opinion in Environmental Science & Health*, 31, 2023, 100413.
7. https://www.newscientist.com/article/mg25834450-800-the-civilisation-myth-how-new-discoveries-are-rewriting-human-history/ — retrieved 15/12/2023
8. https://www.nationalgeographic.com/what-the-world-eats/ — retrieved 22/11/2023
9. https://ourworldindata.org/grapher/share-cereals-animal-feed?time=2020 — retrieved 22/11/2023
10. https://www.newscientist.com/article/2383747-your-genes-may-influence-how-much-fruit-fish-or-salt-you-eat/ — retrieved 22/11/2023
11. https://www.theguardian.com/environment/2011/mar/31/insects-uk-diet-2020 — retrieved 22/11/2023
12. https://en.wikipedia.org/wiki/List_of_countries_by_life_expectancy/ — retrieved 15/12/2023
13. Erlandson, Jon M., Todd J. Braje, Kristina M. Gill, and Michael H. Graham. 'Ecology of the Kelp Highway: Did Marine Resources Facilitate Human Dispersal From Northeast Asia

to the Americas?', *The Journal of Island and Coastal Archaeology*, 10(3), 2015, pp. 392-411, DOI: 10.1080/15564894.2014.1001923

14 Erlandson, Jon M., Michael H. Graham, Bruce J. Bourque, Debra Corbett, James A. Estes, and Robert S. Steneck. 'The Kelp Highway Hypothesis: Marine Ecology, the Coastal Migration Theory, and the Peopling of the Americas', *The Journal of Island and Coastal Archaeology*, 2(2), 2007, pp. 161-74.

15 https://www.newscientist.com/article/dn25575-flooded-cave-hides-naia-a-13000-year-old-american/ — retrieved 17/12/2023

16 Dillehay, T., and M. Collins. 'Early cultural evidence from Monte Verde in Chile', *Nature*, 332, 1988, pp. 150-52.

17 Kareklas, K., D. Nettle, and T.V. Smulders. 'Water-induced finger wrinkles improve handling of wet objects', *Biology Letters*, 9(2), 2013, 20120999.

18 Changizi, M., R. Weber, R. Kotecha, and J. Palazzo. 'Are wet-induced wrinkled fingers primate rain treads?', *Brain, Behavior and Evolution*, 77(4), 2011, pp. 286-90. https://doi.org/10.1159/000328223

19 Kumar, N. 'Soil Degradation and its Causes', *International Journal For Multidisciplinary Research*, 5(1), 2023. https://doi.org/10.36948/ijfmr.2023.v05i01.1443

20 Goulart, H. M. D., K. van der Wiel, C. Folberth, J. Balkovic, and B. van den Hurk. 'Storylines of weather-induced crop failure events under climate change', *Earth System Dynamics*, 12(4), 2021, pp. 1503-27. https://doi.org/10.5194/esd-12-1503-2021

21 Zurek, Monika, Aniek Hebinck, and Odirilwe Selomane. 'Looking across diverse food system futures: Implications for climate change and the environment', *Q Open*, 1(1), 2021, qoaa001. https://doi.org/10.1093/qopen/qoaa001

22 https://www.greenwave.org/ — retrieved 18/12/2023

23 https://www.newyorker.com/magazine/2015/11/02/a-new-leaf

24 https://gallowaywildfoods.com/foraged-dashi-broth-with-reedmace-and-spoot-clams/ — retrieved 18/12/2023
25 https://gallowaywildfoods.com/product/recorded-webinar-a-foragers-guide-to-seaweeds/ — retrieved 18/12/2023
26 https://www.ciwf.org.uk/factory-farming/animal-cruelty/ — retrieved 18/12/2023
27 https://www.theguardian.com/lifeandstyle/2021/may/27/accidental-meat-should-carnivores-embrace-eating-roadkill — retrieved 18/12/2023
28 https://www.theguardian.com/society/2023/mar/17/deer-destroying-habitats-venison-uk-food-banks — retrieved 18/12/2023
29 https://forestrycommission.blog.gov.uk/2022/08/04/reducing-the-impact-of-deer-on-the-natural-environment-consultation-opens/ — retrieved 18/12/2023
30 https://www.sciencedaily.com/releases/2024/02/240214203323.htm — retrieved 16/7/2024
31 https://www.imdb.com/title/tt13648824/ — retrieved 18/12/2023
32 https://youtu.be/pnuzEbz4hXw?feature=shared&t=20 — read the comments below the video! — retrieved 19/12/2023
33 https://www.youtube.com/watch?v=vLJ9i055pGE — retrieved 18/12/2023
34 https://monicawilde.com/the-wildbiome-project-results/ — retrieved 18/12/2023
35 https://www.legislation.gov.uk/ukpga/1991/54/section/4 — retrieved 18/12/2023
36 Fajzel, W., E.D. Galbraith, C. Barrington-Leigh, J. Charmes, E. Frie, I. Hatton, P. Le Mézo, R. Milo, K. Minor, X. Wan, V. Xia, and S. Xu. 'The global human day', *Proceedings of the National Academy of Sciences of the United States of America*, 120(25), 2023, e2219564120. https://doi.org/10.1073/pnas.2219564120

Chapter Two: Consciousness

1. https://www.verywellmind.com/what-meditating-every-day-does-to-your-brain-8656065 — retrieved 16/7/2024
2. https://www.sciencemuseum.org.uk/objects-and-stories/medicine/medicine-aftermath-war — retrieved 25/1/2023
3. https://www.defensemedianetwork.com/stories/treatment-war-related-psychiatric-injuries-post-world-war-ii/ — retrieved 27/1/2023
4. https://www.bbc.com/travel/article/20201101-the-truth-about-british-stoicism — retrieved 28/6/2023
5. Möller, E.L., M. Majdandžić, and S.M. Bögels. 'Parental anxiety, parenting behavior, and infant anxiety: differential associations for fathers and mothers', *Journal of Child and Family Studies*, 24(9), 2015, pp. 2626–37. https://doi.org/10.1007/s10826-014-0065-7
6. https://www.nature.com/articles/31719 1a0.pdf — retrieved 28/6/2023
7. Cohen, Emily Wanderer. *From Generation to Generation*. Morgan James Publishing, 2018.
8. Feeney, Kevin M. *Fly Agaric: a compendium of history, pharmacology, mythology and exploration*. Fly Agaric Press, 2020, p. 102.
9. NIOZ Royal Netherlands Institute for Sea Research. 'Greening of Sahara desert triggered early human migrations out of Africa', *ScienceDaily*, 2009, www.sciencedaily.com/releases/2009/11/091111115843.htm — retrieved 18/5/2021
10. Zeng, T.C., A.J. Aw, and M.W. Feldman. 'Cultural hitchhiking and competition between patrilineal kin groups explain the post-Neolithic Y-chromosome bottleneck', *Nature Communications*, 9(1), 2018, 2077. https://doi.org/10.1038/s41467-018-04375-6

11 Penezić, Kristina, Marko Porčić, Petra Kathrin Urban, Ursula Wittwer-Backofen, and Sofija Stefanović. 'Stressful times for women – Increased physiological stress in Neolithic females detected in tooth cementum', *Journal of Archaeological Science*, 122, 2020, 105217, ISSN 0305-4403 https://doi.org/10.1016/j.jas.2020.105217

12 Fukuda, Misao, and Kiyomi Fukuda. 'The male to female ratio of newborn infants in Japan in relation to climate change, earthquakes, fetal deaths, and singleton male and female birth weights', *Early Human Development*, 140, 2020, 104861, ISSN 0378-3782

13 Masukume G., M. Ryan, R. Masukume, D. Zammit, V. Grech, and W. Mapanga. 'COVID-19 onset reduced the sex ratio at birth in South Africa', *PeerJ*, 10, 2022, e13985

14 Mckenna, T. *Food of the Gods: the search for the original tree of knowledge: a radical history of plants, drugs and human evolution.* Bantam, 1993.

15 Ruiz-Almenara, C., E. Gándara, and M. Gómez-Hernández, M. 'Comparison of diversity and composition of macrofungal species between intensive mushroom harvesting and non-harvesting areas in Oaxaca, Mexico', *PeerJ*, 7, 2019, e8325

16 Muttoni, S., M. Ardissino, and C. John. 'Classical psychedelics for the treatment of depression and anxiety: A systematic review', *Journal of Affective Disorders*, 258, 2019, pp. 11–24.

17 DiVito, A.J., and R.F. Leger. 'Psychedelics as an emerging novel intervention in the treatment of substance use disorder: a review', *Molecular Biology Reports*, 47(12), 2020, pp. 9791–99.

18 Cherian, K.N., J.N. Keynan, L. Anker, et al. 'Magnesium-ibogaine therapy in veterans with traumatic brain injuries', *Nature Medicine*, 30, 2024, pp. 373–81. https://doi.org/10.1038/s41591-023-02705-w

19 http://news.bbc.co.uk/1/hi/uk/4691899.stm — retrieved 17/2/2023
20 Carhart-Harris R.L., M. Bolstridge, J. Rucker, C.M. Day, D. Erritzoe, M. Kaelen, M. Bloomfield, J.A. Rickard, B. Forbes, A. Feilding, D. Taylor, S. Pilling, V.H. Curran, D.J. Nutt. 'Psilocybin with psychological support for treatment-resistant depression: an open-label feasibility study', Lancet Psychiatry. 3(7), 2016, pp. 619–27. DOI: 10.1016/S2215-0366(16)30065-7
21 https://www.bbc.co.uk/news/health-56745139 — retrieved 17/2/2023
22 https://www.psychologytoday.com/us/blog/balanced/202007/magic-mushrooms-and-the-future-psychology retrieved 17/2/2023
23 https://www.independent.co.uk/life-style/health-and-families/magic-mushrooms-chemical-depression-help-treat-psychiatrist-name-any-key-science-terms-names-etc-a7739941.html retrieved 17/2/2023
24 https://www.youtube.com/watch?v=MqfC9bRY3CI — retrieved 17/2/2023
25 https://www.youtube.com/watch?v=99B-BRT1dqI — retrieved 8/7/2024
26 https://www.youtube.com/watch?v=qzgtJleG3r8 — retrieved 8/7/2024
27 Pollan, Michael. *How to Change Your Mind: the new science of psychedelics.* Penguin Books, 2018.
28 https://www.youtube.com/watch?v=UYAy4G1i0As — retrieved 9/7/2024
29 https://www.youtube.com/watch?v=-sk6Vd9OGdE — retrieved 31/10/2022
30 https://www.verywellmind.com/understanding-ocd-and-stress-2510559 — retrieved 5/7/2023

31 Bartkowski, J., G. Acevedo, and H. van Loggerenberg. 'Prayer, Meditation, and Anxiety: Durkheim Revisited', *Religions*, 8(9), 2017, p. 191. https://doi.org/10.3390/rel8090191

32 Rahayu, I.N., L. Diana, and R.V.Y. Tjahjono. 'Effects of Morning's Prayer Routines in The Congregation on Random Blood Sugar Levels of Elderly at Al Wahyu Mosque Rungkut Surabaya', *Oceana Biomedicina Journal*, 4(2), 2021, pp. 133-44. https://doi.org/10.30649/obj.v4i2.12

33 Mather, Maraa, Nichole R. Lighthall, Lina Nga, and Marissa A. Gorlick. 'Sex differences in how stress affects brain activity during face viewing', *NeuroReport*, 21(14), 2010, pp. 933-37. DOI: 10.1097/WNR.0b013e32833ddd92

34 https://www.ancientpages.com/2019/10/03/utiseta-norse-vision-quest-ancient-spiritual-tradition-of-northern-europe/ — retrieved 8/07/2024

35 Stephenson, B. (2003). Ritual criticism of a contemporary rite of passage. *Journal of Ritual Studies*, 17(1), 32-41. http://www.jstor.org/stable/44368643

36 https://simple.wikipedia.org/wiki/Vision_quest#:~:text=A%20vision%20quest%20was%20a,provide%20wisdom%2C%20protection%20or%20advice — retrieved 8/7/2024

37 Shaw, M. and L. Cooper. *Wolf Milk: chthonic memory in the deep wild*. Cista Mystica, 2019.

38 Divya, R., V. Ashok, and M. Rajajeyakumar. 'Nomophobia: The Invisible Addiction', *Psychology and Behavioral Science International Journal*, 10(5), 2019, 555799. https://doi.org/10.19080/pbsij.2019.10.555799

39 Farooqui, I.A., P. Pore, and J. Gothankar. 'Nomophobia: an emerging issue in medical institutions?', *Journal of Mental Health*, 27(5), 2017, pp. 438-41. https://doi.org/10.1080/09638237.2017.1417564

40 Rodríguez-García, A-M., A-J. Moreno-Guerrero, and J. López Belmonte. 'Nomophobia: An Individual's Growing Fear of Being without a Smartphone—A Systematic Literature Review', *International Journal of Environmental Research and Public Health*, 17(2), 2020, 580. https://doi.org/10.3390/ijerph17020580

41 https://www.uswitch.com/mobiles/studies/mobile-statistics/ — retrieved 8/7/2024

42 https://www.gsma.com/newsroom/press-release/smartphone-owners-are-now-the-global-majority-new-gsma-report-reveals/ — retrieved 8/7/2024

43 Weiste, Elina, Miira Niska, Taina Valkeapää, and Melisa Stevanovic. 'Goal Setting in Mental Health Rehabilitation: References to Competence and Interest as Resources for Negotiating Goals', *Journal of Psychosocial Rehabilitation and Mental Health*, 9, 2022, pp. 409-24. https://doi.org/10.1007/s40737-022-00280-w

44 Park H.Y., E. Seo, K.M. Park, S.J. Koo, E. Lee, and S.K. An. 'Shame and guilt in youth at ultra-high risk for psychosis', *Comprehensive Psychiatry*, 108, 2021, 152241. DOI: 10.1016/j.comppsych.2021.152241

45 Rees, W.D. 'The Hallucinations of Widowhood', *British Medical Journal*, 4, 1971, p. 37. DOI: 10.1136/bmj.4.5778.37

46 https://www.rcpsych.ac.uk/docs/default-source/members/sigs/spirituality-spsig/spirituality-special-interest-group-publications-nicki-crowley-psychosis-or-spiritual-emergence.pdf?sfvrsn=5685d4c1_2 — retrieved 3/7/2023

47 Jonsson, G., and E. Nwanze. 'Selective (+)-Amphetamine Neurotoxicity on Striatal Dopamine Nerve Terminals in the Mouse', *British Journal of Pharmacology*, 77(2), 1982, pp. 335-345. https://doi.org/10.1111/j.1476-5381.1982.tb09303.x

48 Kelleher, I., D. Connor, M.C. Clarke, N. Devlin, M. Harley,

49. Krasskova, G., and R. Kaldera. *Northern Tradition for the Solitary Practitioner*. Red Wheel/Weiser, 2008.
50. Exodus 34:28. 'He was there with the LORD forty days and forty nights; he neither ate bread, nor drank water. He wrote on the tablets the words of the covenant, the ten commandments.'
51. Matthew 4:1. 'Then Jesus was led by the Spirit into the wilderness to be tempted by the devil. After fasting forty days and forty nights, he was hungry.'
52. يَٰٓأَيُّهَا ٱلَّذِينَ ءَامَنُوا۟ كُتِبَ عَلَيْكُمُ ٱلصِّيَامُ كَمَا كُتِبَ عَلَى ٱلَّذِينَ مِن قَبْلِكُمْ لَعَلَّكُمْ تَتَّقُونَ ١٨٣ 'O believers! Fasting is prescribed for you — as it was for those before you — so perhaps you will become mindful of Allah.'
53. https://www.livescience.com/who-was-siddhartha-gautama-the-buddha — retrieved 3/7/2023
54. McBride, R.D. 'The Vision-Quest Motif in Narrative Literature on the Buddhist Traditions of Silla', *Korean Studies*, 27, 2003, pp. 16–47. http://www.jstor.org/stable/23719569
55. https://www.rcpsych.ac.uk/docs/default-source/members/sigs/spirituality-spsig/spirituality-special-interest-group-publications-nicki-crowley-psychosis-or-spiritual-emergence.pdf?sfvrsn=5685d4c1_2 — normalisation retrieved 3/7/2023
56. *Crataegus monogyna*
57. *Aegopodium podagraria*
58. *Daucus carota*
59. *Ficaria verna*
60. *Rumex obtusifolius*

61 *Taraxacum officinale*
62 *Sinapis arvensis*
63 *Bellis perennis*
64 *Cardamine hirsuta*
65 https://en.wikipedia.org/wiki/Magic_circle — retrieved 3/7/2023
66 https://youtu.be/PovPsoVl7hw?t=10 — retrieved 3/7/2023
67 http://www.newforestexplorersguide.co.uk/wildlife/mammals/foxes/family-life.html — retrieved 3/7/2023
68 Hanevik, H., K.A. Hestad, L. Lien, I. Joa, T.K. Larsen, and L.J. Danbolt. 'Religiousness in First-Episode Psychosis', *Archiv Für Religionspsychologie / Archive for the Psychology of Religion*, 39(2), 2017, pp. 139–64. http://www.jstor.org/stable/26379582

Chapter Three: Shelter

1 Anthes, E. *The Great Indoors*. Scientific American / Farrar, Straus and Giroux, 2020.
2 https://www.ons.gov.uk/employmentandlabourmarket/peopleinwork/employmentandemployeetypes/articles/characteristicsofhomeworkersgreatbritain/september2022tojanuary2023 — retrieved 8/7/2024
3 https://www.worldhealth.net/news/impact-remote-work-weight-and-obesity-older-adults/ — retrieved 9/7/2024
4 Kallestad, Håvard, Henrik B. Jacobsen, Nils Inge Landrø, Petter C. Borchgrevink, and Tore C. Stiles. 'The role of insomnia in the treatment of chronic fatigue', *Journal of Psychosomatic Research*, 78(5), 2015, pp. 427–32, ISSN 0022-3999
5 Li, Q., H. Ochiai, T. Ochiai, N. Takayama, S. Kumeda, T. Miura, Y. Aoyagi, and M. Imai. 'Effects of forest bathing (shinrin-yoku) on serotonin in serum, depressive symptoms and subjective sleep quality in middle-aged males',

Environmental Health and Preventive Medicine, 27, 2022, p. 44. https://doi.org/10.1265/ehpm.22-00136

6 Horiuchi, M., J. Endo, S. Akatsuka, T. Hasegawa, E. Yamamoto, T. Uno, and S. Kikuchi. 'An effective strategy to reduce blood pressure after forest walking in middle-aged and aged people'. *Journal of Physical Therapy Science*, 27(12), 2015, pp. 3711–16. https://doi.org/10.1589/jpts.27.3711

7 Tsao, T-M., M-J. Tsai, J-S. Hwang, W-F. Cheng, C-F. Wu, C-C.K. Chou, and T-C. Su. 'Health effects of a forest environment on natural killer cells in humans: an observational pilot study', *Oncotarget*, 9(23), 2018, pp. 16501–11. https://doi.org/10.18632/oncotarget.24741

8 https://qxmd.com/calculate/calculator_146/hamilton-depression-rating-scale-ham-d-or-hdrs# — retrieved 31/8/2023

9 Hidaka, B. H. 'Depression as a disease of modernity: explanations for increasing prevalence', *Journal of Affective Disorders*, 140(3), 2012, pp. 205–14. https://doi.org/10.1016/j.jad.2011.12.036

10 Barton, J., and M. Rogerson. 'The importance of greenspace for mental health', *British Journal of Psychiatry International*, 14(4), 2017, pp. 79–81. DOI: 10.1192/s2056474000002051. PMID: 29093955; PMCID: PMC5663018

11 https://historicengland.org.uk/whats-new/debate/recent/public-parks/the-victorian-legacy/ — retrieved 1/9/2023

12 Hewitt, Robert. 'The Influence of Somatic and Psychiatric Medical Theory on the Design of Nineteenth Century American Cities', *Priory Lodge Education Ltd.*, 2003. https://www.priory.com/homol/19c.htm

13 Olmsted, Frederick Law. 'Public Parks and the Enlargement of Towns', read before the American Social Science Association at the Lowell Institute, Boston, 1870, in Beverage, Charles E.

and Carolyn Hoffman, eds, *The Papers of Frederick Law Olmsted, Supplementary Series I, Writings on Public Parks, Parkways, and Park Systems*, The Johns Hopkins University Press, 1997, p. 187.
14 Pretty, J. *Agri-Culture Reconnecting People, Land and Nature*. Routledge, 2013.
15 ---. *Smoke Hole: Looking to the Wild in the Time of the Spyglass*. White River Junction, Vermont, Chelsea Green Publishing, 2021.
16 Li, Qing. *Shinrin-Yoku*. Penguin, 2018.
17 Hartig, T., R. Catalano, M. Ong, and S.L. Syme. 'Vacation, Collective Restoration, and Mental Health in a Population', *Society and Mental Health*, 3(3), 2013, pp. 221–36. https://doi.org/10.1177/2156869313497718
18 https://www.bbc.co.uk/news/uk-england-tyne-64841784 — retrieved 1/9/2023
19 Talman, C.F. 'The Elusive Will-o'-the Wisp', *Scientific American*, 74(1907supp), 1912, pp. 47–8. https://doi.org/10.1038/scientificamerican07201912-47supp
20 Li, Y., G. Li, L. Liu, and H. Wu. 'Correlations between mobile phone addiction and anxiety, depression, impulsivity, and poor sleep quality among college students: A systematic review and meta-analysis', *Journal of Behavioral Addictions*, 9(3), 2020, pp. 551–71. https://doi.org/10.1556/2006.2020.00057
21 Wach, K., C.D. Duong, J. Eidys, R. Kazlauskaitė, P. Korzynski, G. Mazurek, J. Paliszkiewicz & E. Ziemba. 'The dark side of generative artificial intelligence: A critical analysis of controversies and risks of ChatGPT'. *Entrepreneurial Business and Economics Review*, 11(2), 2023, pp. 7–30.
22 Kaplan, R., and S. Kaplan. *The Experience of Nature: a psychological perspective*. Cambridge University Press, 1989.
23 https://en.wikipedia.org/wiki/Directed_attention_fatigue — retrieved 4/9/2023

24. Kaplan S., and M.G. Berman. 'Directed Attention as a Common Resource for Executive Functioning and Self-Regulation', *Perspectives on Psychological Science*, 5(1), 2010, pp. 43–57.
25. https://www.mentalhealth.org.uk/explore-mental-health/statistics/anxiety-statistics — retrieved 6/9/2023
26. https://www.statista.com/statistics/1132658/anxiety-symptoms-us-adults-by-date-past-week/ — retrieved 6/9/2023
27. Jung, C. G., and Meredith Sabini. *The Earth Has a Soul: C.G. Jung on Nature, Technology & Modern Life*. Berkeley, California, North Atlantic Books, 2016.
28. https://www.theguardian.com/education/2002/apr/22/highereducation.globalisation — retrieved 12/08/2024
29. https://news.sanfordhealth.org/heart/sitting-is-the-new-smoking-truly-a-silent-killer/ — retrieved 26/7/2023
30. Wadley, Lyn. et al. 'Middle Stone Age Bedding Construction and Settlement Patterns at Sibudu, South Africa', *Science*, 334, 2011, pp. 1388–91. DOI: 10.1126/science.1213317
31. https://www.tshaonline.org/handbook/entries/hinds-cave-site — retrieved 29/7/2023
32. https://www.thespruce.com/the-history-of-the-bed-4062296 — retrieved 29/7/2023
33. https://en.wikipedia.org/wiki/File:Harp_player,_Cycladic_civilization_-_Greece.JPG — retrieved 31/7/2023
34. https://www.theatlantic.com/international/archive/2016/08/chairs-history-witold-rybczynski/497657/ — retrieved 31/7/2023
35. Bowman, K. *Rethink Your Position*. Propriometrics Press, 2023.
36. Coenen, P., S. Parry, L. Willenberg, J.W. Shi, L. Romero, D.M. Blackwood, G.N. Healy, D.W. Dunstan, L.M. Straker. 'Associations of prolonged standing with musculoskeletal symptoms – a systematic review of laboratory studies', *Gait*

Posture, 58, 2017, pp. 310–18. DOI: 10.1016/j.gaitpost.2017.08.024
37   Steward, Julian H. *Handbook of South American Indians, Vol. 5.* Forgotten Books, 2017.
38   Barnhouse, Rebecca. *The Old English Hexateuch.* Medieval Institute Publications, 2000.
39   https://www.newscientist.com/lastword/mg24432561-400-sitting-pretty-sitting-is-harmful-but-how-exactly-is-it-bad/ – retrieved 26/7/2023
40   Dunn, K.M., L. Hestbaek, J.D. Cassidy. 'Low back pain across the life course', *Best Practice and Research Clinical Rheumatology*, 27(5), 2013, pp. 591–600.
41   Shiri, Rahman, et al., 'The Association Between Obesity and Low Back Pain: A Meta-Analysis', *American Journal of Epidemiology*, 171(2), 2010, pp. 135–54, https://doi.org/10.1093/aje/kwp356
42   https://www.healthline.com/health/how-long-does-it-take-to-form-a-habit#psychology-behind-it – retrieved 14/7/2023
43   https://www.gov.uk/child-car-seats-the-rules – retrieved 18/7/2023. Children must normally use a child car seat until they're 12 years old or 135 centimetres tall, whichever comes first.
44   Kim, Y., H. Kang, S. Kim, and K. Park. 'Prolonged sitting-induced back pain influences abdominal muscle thickness in a sitting but not a supine position', *Scientific Reports*, 11(1), 2021, 16369. https://doi.org/10.1038/s41598-021-95795-w
45   Hewes, G.W. 'World Distribution of Certain Postural Habits', *American Anthropologist*, 57(2), 1955, pp. 231–44. http://www.jstor.org/stable/666393
46   Patel, Alpa V., et al., 'Leisure Time Spent Sitting in Relation to Total Mortality in a Prospective Cohort of US Adults', *American Journal of Epidemiology*, 172(4), 2010, pp. 419–29,

https://doi.org/10.1093/aje/kwq155
47 https://youtu.be/VH0TANG0q-w — hammock
48 https://youtu.be/UV9t5jCHkJc — chair
49 Bontrup, Carolin, William R. Taylor, Michael Fliesser, Rosa Visscher, Tamara Green, Pia-Maria Wippert, and Roland Zemp. 'Low back pain and its relationship with sitting behaviour among sedentary office workers', *Applied Ergonomics*, 81, 2019, 102894, ISSN 0003-6870
50 Bauman, A.E., J.Y. Chau, D. Ding, and J. Bennie. 'Too much sitting and cardio-metabolic risk: an update of epidemiological evidence', *Current Cardiovascular Risk Reports*, 7(4), 2013, pp. 293–8. https://doi.org/10.1007/s12170-013-0316-y
51 Lurati, A.R. 'Health Issues and Injury Risks Associated With Prolonged Sitting and Sedentary Lifestyles', *Workplace Health & Safety*, 66(6), 2018, pp. 285–90.

Chapter Four: Bodies

1 Fajzel, W., E.D. Galbraith, C. Barrington-Leigh, J. Charmes, E. Frie, I. Hatton, P. Le Mézo, R. Milo, K. Minor, X. Wan, V. Xia, and S. Xu. 'The global human day', *Proceedings of the National Academy of Sciences of the United States of America*, 120(25), 2023, e2219564120. https://doi.org/10.1073/pnas.2219564120
2 Cecchetto, Cinzia, Elisa Dal Bò, Emma T. Eliasson, Elisa Vigna, Ludovica Natali, Enzo Pasquale Scilingo, Alberto Greco, Fabio Di Francesco, Gergö Hadlaczky, Johan N. Lundström, Vladimir Carli, and Claudio Gentili. 'Sniffing Out a Solution: Emotional Body Odors Can Improve Mindfulness Therapy for Social Anxiety Symptoms But Not for Depressive Symptoms', 2023. Available at SSRN: https://ssrn.com/abstract=4591481 or http://dx.doi.org/10.2139/ssrn.4591481
3 Caress, S.M., and A.C. Steinemann. 'Prevalence of fragrance

sensitivity in the American population', *Journal of Environmental Health*, 71(7), 2009, pp. 46–50. PMID: 19326669.

4 Fukutomi, Y., M. Taniguchi, H. Nakamura, and K. Akiyama. 'Epidemiological link between wheat allergy and exposure to hydrolyzed wheat protein in facial soap', *Allergy*, 69(10), 2014, pp. 1405–11. https://onlinelibrary.wiley.com/doi/10.1111/all.12481

5 McDonald, Brian C., et al. 'Volatile chemical products emerging as largest petrochemical source of urban organic emissions', *Science*, 359, 2018, pp. 76-4. DOI: 10.1126/science.aaq0524

6 https://www.theguardian.com/society/2021/sep/27/covid-has-wiped-out-years-of-progress-on-life-expectancy-finds-study — retrieved 16/12/2021

7 https://www.cdc.gov/nchs/pressroom/podcasts/2021/20210721/20210721.htm — retrieved 16/12/2021

8 https://www.ncbi.nlm.nih.gov/pmc/articles/PMC6048199/ — retrieved 17/12/2021

9 https://news.harvard.edu/gazette/story/2020/07/the-hair-raising-reason-for-goosebumps-is-revealed/ — retrieved 20/2/2022

10 Thorstenson, Christopher A., Adam D. Pazda and Stephanie Lichtenfeld. 'Facial blushing influences perceived embarrassment and related social functional evaluations', *Cognition and Emotion*, 34:3, 2020, pp. 413–26, DOI: 10.1080/02699931.2019.1634004

11 Montgomery, Doil D. *Encyclopedia of Psychotherapy*, 2002, pp. 331–44.

12 https://www.theguardian.com/environment/2016/mar/25/three-quarters-of-uk-children-spend-less-time-outdoors-than-prison-inmates-survey — retrieved 19/1/2022

13 Palmer, D.J. 'Vitamin D and the Development of Atopic

Eczema', *Journal of Clinical Medicine*, 4(5), 2015, pp. 1036–50. DOI: 10.3390/jcm4051036, https://www.ncbi.nlm.nih.gov/pmc/articles/PMC4470215/

14 https://patient.info/skin-conditions/atopic-eczema/eczema-triggers-and-irritants#nav-1 — retrieved 31/1/2022

15 I must point out that the reasons for this rise, along with the rise in other autoimmune conditions, like lupus and Crohn's disease, are not all the fault of indoor bathrooms alone. Dr Moncrieff suggests that there is a link between overuse of antibiotics in children and the rising rates of eczema and asthma. Also, researchers James Lee and Carola Vinuesa from London's Francis Crick Institute point the finger at fast-food diets. Suffering from two autoimmune conditions myself, I think it's a vicious cocktail of factors that includes antibiotics, stress, loneliness, and perhaps even the hum of traffic noise.

16 https://www.youtube.com/watch?v=jzYDVQ_ECyU — retrieved 21/1/2022

17 Routh, Hirak Behari, Kazal Rekha Bhowmik, Lawrence Charles Parish, and Joseph A. Witkowski. 'Soaps: From the phoenicians to the 20th century — A historical review', *Clinics in Dermatology*, 14(1), 1996, pp. 3–6, ISSN 0738-081X, https://doi.org/10.1016/0738-081X(95)00101-K

18 Draelos, Zoe Diana, 'Cosmetics and Skin Care Products: A Historical Perspective', *Dermatologic Clinics*, 18(4), 2000, pp. 557–9, ISSN 0733-8635, https://doi.org/10.1016/S0733-8635(05)70206-0

19 Te Hennepe, M. '"To Preserve the Skin in Health": Drainage, Bodily Control and the Visual Definition of Healthy Skin 1835–1900', *Medical History*, 58(3), 2014, pp. 397–421. DOI: 10.1017/mdh.2014.30

20 Hamblin, J. *Clean*. Penguin, 2020.

21 https://psychcentral.com/blog/life-goals/2018/09/attractive-people-hiring#Beautiful-people-and-the-job-hunt — retrieved 19/1/2022

22 https://news.cornell.edu/stories/2010/05/unattractive-people-pay-price-court — retrieved 19/1/2022

23 https://www.youtube.com/watch?v=JFSVbBW5Cg4 — retrieved 19/1/2022

24 https://www.youtube.com/watch?v=IdmQg3r0S18 — retrieved 19/1/2022

25 Fenga, C., S. Gangemi, and C. Costa. 'Benzene exposure is associated with epigenetic changes (Review)', *Molecular Medicine Reports*, 13, 2016, pp. 3401–5. https://doi.org/10.3892/mmr.2016.4955

26 https://www.wistv.com/story/5250182/study-shampoo-ingredient-may-affect-brain-development/ and https://www.ncbi.nlm.nih.gov/books/NBK373177/ — retrieved 31/1/2022

27 Koniecki, Diane, Rong Wang, Richard P. Moody, and Jiping Zhu. 'Phthalates in cosmetic and personal care products: Concentrations and possible dermal exposure', *Environmental Research*, 111(3), 2011, pp. 329–36, ISSN 0013-9351, https://doi.org/10.1016/j.envres.2011.01.013

28 https://www.newscientist.com/article/mg25333700-100-toxic-chemicals-are-everywhere-in-our-daily-lives-can-we-avoid-them/ — retrieved 19/1/2022

29 https://www.youtube.com/watch?v=FcZsYz7-RYw — retrieved 21/1/2022

30 https://www.ncbi.nlm.nih.gov/pmc/articles/PMC3013594/ — retrieved 24/2/2022

31 A quick note of warning, however: potassium alum is still relatively untested by the scientific peer review process and so it might be that I return to this underarm solution and review it at a later date.

32 Sikirov, D. 'Comparison of straining during defecation in three positions: results and implications for human health', *Digestive Diseases and Sciences*, 48(7), 2003, pp. 1201–5. DOI: 10.1023/a:1024180319005. PMID: 12870773.

33 Enders, Giulia. *Gut: the inside story of our body's most under-rated organ*. Scribe Publications, 2017.

34 http://news.bbc.co.uk/1/hi/health/1399412.stm — retrieved 10/12/2021

35 https://www.timeout.com/movies/the-young-offenders — retrieved 9/12/2021

36 https://washingtoncitypaper.com/article/191664/when-and-why-did-humans-start-wiping-or-manually-cleaning-themselves-postdefecation/ — retrieved 9/12/2021

37 https://www.menshealth.com/health/a37667268/what-is-a-ghost-poop/ — retrieved 9/12/2021

38 Charlier, P., L. Brun, C. Prêtre, and I. Huynh-Charlier. 'Toilet hygiene in the classical era', *British Medical Journal*, 345, 2012, e8287. DOI: 10.1136/bmj.e8287

39 https://www.museums.norfolk.gov.uk/-/media/museums/downloads/time-and-tide/x-is-for-xylospongium-checked.pdf — retrieved 1/2/2022

40 https://www-nature-com.plsa2r.idm.oclc.org/articles/533456a — retrieved 1/2/2022

41 https://www.nhs.uk/live-well/sexual-health/keeping-your-vagina-clean-and-healthy/ — retrieved 17/1/2022

42 Song, S.G., and S.H. Kim. 'Pruritus ani', *Journal of the Korean Society of Coloproctology*, 27(2), 2011, pp. 54–7. DOI: 10.3393/jksc.2011.27.2.54

43 Lieberman, D. *Exercised: the science of physical activity, rest and health*. Allen Lane, 2020.

44 Li, H., X. Zhang, S. Bi, H. Liu, Y. Cao, and G. Zhang. 'Green Exercise: Can Nature Video Benefit Isometric Exercise?',

International Journal of Environmental Research and Public Health, 18(11), 2021, 5554. https://doi.org/10.3390/ijerph18115554

45 https://preview.discovermagazine.com/health/gene-mutation-made-our-ancestors-better-long-distance-runners — retrieved 6/7/2022

46 Sato, Hiroyuki, 'Late Pleistocene trap-pit hunting in the Japanese Archipelago', *Quaternary International*, 248, 2012, pp. 43–55, ISSN 1040-6182, https://doi.org/10.1016/j.quaint.2010.11.026

47 Wood, B.M., J.A. Harris, D.A. Raichlen, H. Pontzer, K. Sayre, A. Sancilio, C. Berbesque, A.N. Crittenden, A. Mabulla, R. McElreath, E. Cashdan, and J.H. Jones. 'Gendered movement ecology and landscape use in Hadza hunter-gatherers', *Nature Human Behaviour*, 5(4), 2021, pp. 436–46. https://doi.org/10.1038/s41562-020-01002-7

48 https://www.telegraph.co.uk/news/2020/05/08/pm-urged-allow-gym-reopening-exercise-wonder-drug-coronavirus/ — retrieved 18/3/2022

49 Arem, H., S.C. Moore, A. Patel, P. Hartge, A. Berrington de Gonzalez, K. Visvanathan, P.T. Campbell, M. Freedman, E. Weiderpass, H.O. Adami, M.S. Linet, I.M. Lee, and C.E. Matthews. 'Leisure time physical activity and mortality: a detailed pooled analysis of the dose-response relationship', *JAMA Internal Medicine*, 175(6), 2015, pp. 959–67. https://doi.org/10.1001/jamainternmed.2015.0533

50 O'Donovan, G., I.M. Lee, M. Hamer, and E. Stamatakis. 'Association of "Weekend Warrior" and Other Leisure Time Physical Activity Patterns With Risks for All-Cause, Cardiovascular Disease, and Cancer Mortality', *JAMA Internal Medicine*, 177(3), 2017, pp. 335–342. https://doi.org/10.1001/jamainternmed.2016.8014

51 Williams, Paul T., and Paul D. Thompson. 'Walking Versus Running for Hypertension, Cholesterol, and Diabetes Mellitus Risk Reduction', *Arteriosclerosis, Thrombosis, and Vascular Biology*, 33, 2013, pp. 1085–91. https://doi.org/10.1161/ATVBAHA.112.300878

52 https://www.healthline.com/health/walking-vs-running#summary — retrieved 31/3/2022

53 https://www.bbc.com/future/article/20170612-what-you-can-learn-from-einsteins-quirky-habits — retrieved 30/3/2022

54 https://www.theatlantic.com/magazine/archive/1905/04/thoreaus-journal-part-iv/542109/ — retrieved 12/08/2024

55 Augusto-Oliveira, M., and A. Verkhratsky. 'Lifestyle-dependent microglial plasticity: training the brain guardians', *Biology Direct*, 16(1), 2021, 12. https://doi.org/10.1186/s13062-021-00297-4

56 Cotman, C.W., and N.C. Berchtold. 'Exercise: a behavioral intervention to enhance brain health and plasticity', *Trends in Neurosciences*, 25, 2002, pp. 295–301.

57 Chang, M., P.V. Jonsson, J. Snaedal, S. Bjornsson, J.S. Saczynski, T. Aspelund, G. Eiriksdottir, M.K. Jonsdottir, O.L. Lopez, T.B. Harris, et al. 'The effect of midlife physical activity on cognitive function among older adults: AGES–Reykjavik Study', *Journals of Gerontology Series A: Biological Sciences and Medical Sciences*, 65, 2010, pp. 1369–74.

58 Schneider, H.J., N. Friedrich, J. Klotsche, L. Pieper, M. Nauck, U. John, M. Dörr, S. Felix, H. Lehnert, D. Pittrow, S. Silber, H. Völzke, G.K. Stalla, H. Wallaschofski, and H.U. Wittchen. 'The predictive value of different measures of obesity for incident cardiovascular events and mortality', *The Journal of clinical endocrinology and metabolism*, 95(4), 2010, pp. 1777–85. https://doi.org/10.1210/jc.2009-1584

59 Dacey, M., A. Baltzell, and L. Zaichkowsky. 'Older adults' intrinsic and extrinsic motivation toward physical activity', *American Journal of Health Behavior*, 32(6), 2008, pp. 570–82. https://doi.org/10.5555/ajhb.2008.32.6.570

Chapter Five: Music

1   Cai, Y., W.L. Zijlema, E.P. Sørgjerd, D. Doiron, K. de Hoogh, S. Hodgson, B. Wolffenbuttel, J. Gulliver, A.L. Hansell, M. Nieuwenhuijsen, K. Rahimi, K., and K. Kvaløy. 'Impact of road traffic noise on obesity measures: Observational study of three European cohorts', *Environmental Research*, 191, 2020, 110013. https://doi.org/10.1016/j.envres.2020.110013

2   https://data.worldobesity.org/country/romania-178/#data_trends – retrieved 5/1/2024

3   D'Souza, Jennifer, Jennifer Weuve, Robert D. Brook, Denis A. Evans, Joel D. Kaufman and Sara D. Adar. 'Long-Term Exposures to Urban Noise and Blood Pressure Levels and Control Among Older Adults', *Hypertension*, 78, 2021, pp. 1801–8. https://doi.org/10.1161/HYPERTENSIONAHA.121.17708

4   ibid.

5   https://www.nhm.ac.uk/discover/how-listening-to-bird-song-can-transform-our-mental-health.html – 26/10/2022

6   https://www.youtube.com/watch?v=wk4qT4J_NUM – retrieved 8/1/2024

7   Männer, J. 'When Does the Human Embryonic Heart Start Beating? A Review of Contemporary and Historical Sources of Knowledge about the Onset of Blood Circulation in Man', *Journal of Cardiovascular Development and Disease*, 9(6), 2022, p. 187. https://doi.org/10.3390/jcdd9060187

8   https://www.abdn.ac.uk/news/3732 – retrieved 5/1/2024

9 Asher, M., A.L. Barthel, S.G. Hofmann, H. Okon-Singer, and I.M. Aderka. 'When two hearts beat as one: Heart-rate synchrony in social anxiety disorder', *Behaviour Research and Therapy*, 141, 2021, 103859. https://doi.org/10.1016/j.brat.2021.103859

10 https://www.psychologytoday.com/gb/blog/your-musical-self/201209/which-came-first-music-or-language — retrieved 14/8/2023

11 Sedghi, Nader, and Elvira Brattico. 'Music og evolution (Music and evolution)', in *Mennesket, Kultur, Evolution: Et Biokulturelt Perspektiv*, Aarhus University Press, 2019, pp. 200–212.

12 Eleuteri, Vesta, et al. 'The Form and Function of Chimpanzee Buttress Drumming', *Animal Behaviour*, 192, 2022, pp. 189–205. https://doi.org/10.1016/j.anbehav.2022.07.013

13 https://www.newscientist.com/article/2167242-how-an-amazonian-people-convey-their-entire-language-by-drumbeat/ — retrieved 8/1/2024

14 https://www.theguardian.com/media/2008/may/21/radio.military — retrieved 8/1/2024

15 Massimello, F., L. Billeci, A. Canu, M.M. Montt-Guevara, G. Impastato, M. Varanini, A. Giannini, T. Simoncini, and P. Mannella, P. 'Music Modulates Autonomic Nervous System Activity in Human Fetuses', *Frontiers in Medicine*, 9, 2022. https://doi.org/10.3389/fmed.2022.857591.

16 Zentner, M., and T. Eerola. 'Rhythmic engagement with music in infancy', *Proceedings of the National Academy of Sciences of the United States of America*, 107(13), 2010, pp. 5768–73. https://doi.org/10.1073/pnas.1000121107

17 Provasi, J., and A. Bobin-Bègue. (2003). 'Spontaneous motor tempo and rhythmical synchronisation in 2½- and 4-year-old children', *International Journal of Behavioral Development*, 27(3), 2003, pp. 220–31.

18 Launay, J., Tarr, B. and Dunbar, R.I.M. (2016), Synchrony as an Adaptive Mechanism for Large-Scale Human Social Bonding. Ethology, 122: 779-789. https://doi.org/10.1111/eth.12528 ps://doi.org/10.1080/01650250244000290

19 https://www.tes.com/magazine/archive/teachers-and-pupils-agree-what-makes-doss-lesson — retrieved 9/7/2024

20 https://www.theatlantic.com/health/archive/2016/03/can-three-words-turn-anxiety-into-success/474909/? — retrieved 2/10/2023

21 Maier, H. 'Rhythmicity — A Powerful Force For Experiencing Unity and Personal Connections', *Journal of Child and Youth Care Work*, 8, 1992, pp. 7–13.

22 Eriksson, C. 'Adlerian Psychology and Music Therapy: The Harmony of Sound and Matter and Community Feeling', *The Journal of Individual Psychology*, 73(3), 2018, pp. 243–64. https://doi.org/10.1353/jip.2017.0020

23 Ascenso, Sara, Rosie Perkins, Louise Atkins, Daisy Fancourt, and Aaron Williamon. 'Promoting well-being through group drumming with mental health service users and their carers', *International Journal of Qualitative Studies on Health and Well-being*, 13(1), 2018. DOI: 10.1080/17482631.2018.1484219

24 https://www.cqc.org.uk/location/RVN2A/reports — retrieved 2/10/2023

25 Winkelman, Michael. 'Complementary Therapy for Addiction: "Drumming Out Drugs"', *American Journal of Public Health*, 93, 2003, pp. 647–51. https://doi.org/10.2105/AJPH.93.4.647

26 https://www.youtube.com/watch?v=5wDFpRgK9WM — retrieved 2/10/2022

27 https://www.youtube.com/watch?v=1tvreQ3hTvA — retrieved 2/10/2022

28 Kjellgren, A., and A. Eriksson, A. 'Altered states during shamanic drumming: A phenomenological study', *International Journal of Transpersonal Studies*, 29(2), 2010, pp. 1-10.

29 Neher, A. (1962). 'A Physiological Explanation of Unusual Behavior in Ceremonies Involving Drums', *Human Biology*, 34(2), 1962, pp. 151-60. http://www.jstor.org/stable/41448545

30 Pekala, R.J. 'The Phenomenology of Consciousness Inventory', in *Quantifying Consciousness: an empirical approach*. Springer, 1991. https://doi.org/10.1007/978-1-4899-0629-8_8

31 Maurer, Sr. Ronald L., V. K. Kumar Ph.D., Lisa Woodside and Ronald J. Pekala. 'Phenomenological Experience in Response to Monotonous Drumming and Hypnotizability', *American Journal of Clinical Hypnosis*, 40(2), 1997, pp. 130-45, DOI: 10.1080/00029157.1997.10403417

32 https://www.youtube.com/watch?v=mFRDhgVs-1Q — retrieved 25/8/2022

33 Cahart, M.S., A. Amad, S.B. Draper, R.G. Lowry, L. Marino, C. Carey, C.E. Ginestet, M.S. Smith, and S.C.R. Williams. 'The effect of learning to drum on behavior and brain function in autistic adolescents', *Proceedings of the National Academy of Sciences of the United States of America*, 119(23), 2022, e2106244119. DOI: 10.1073/pnas.2106244119

34 https://www.youtube.com/watch?v=4lnmNY2ikG4 — retrieved 25/8/2022

35 https://oldtimemusic.com/the-meaning-behind-the-song-hobart-paving-by-saint-etienne/ — retrieved 12/1/2024

36 Cotter, K.N., A.N. Prince, A.P. Christensen, and P.J. Silvia. 'Feeling Like Crying When Listening to Music: Exploring Musical and Contextual Features', *Empirical Studies of the Arts*, 37(2), 2018, pp. 119-37

37 Mayr, Ernst. *What Evolution Is*. Basic Books, 2001, p. 48.

38 https://www.theattic.space/home-page-blogs/2021/1/8/the-woman-who-defied-darwin — retrieved 12/1/2024
39 Darwin, Charles. *The Descent of Man*. (1871). Dover Publications, 2010.
40 Suzuki, T.N. 'Semantic communication in birds: evidence from field research over the past two decades', *Ecological Research*, 31, 2016, pp. 307–19. https://doi.org/10.1007/s11284-016-1339-x
41 Levitin, Daniel J. *This Is Your Brain on Music: the science of a human obsession*. Paw Prints, 2008.
42 Shintel, H. 'Music as Auditory Cheesecake', in: Shackelford, T.K., and V.A. Weekes-Shackelford, eds, *Encyclopedia of Evolutionary Psychological Science*, Springer, 2021. https://doi.org/10.1007/978-3-319-19650-3_2851
43 Sperber, D. *Explaining Culture: a naturalistic approach*. Blackwell, 2002.
44 https://www.statista.com/statistics/1006502/global-population-ten-thousand-bc-to-2050/ — retrieved 12/1/2024
45 Reid, Cornelius L. *Bel Canto: principles and practices*. J. Patelson Music House, 1950.
46 Killin, A. 'The origins of music: Evidence, theory, and prospects', *Music & Science*, 1, 2018. https://doi.org/10.1177/2059204317751971
47 https://time.com/5295907/discover-fire/ — retrieved 13/1/2024
48 https://www.nationalgeographic.com/culture/article/140421-neanderthal-dna-genes-human-ancestry-science — retrieved 13/1/2024
49 Diedrich, Cajus G. '"Neanderthal bone flutes": simply products of Ice Age spotted hyena scavenging activities on cave bear cubs in European cave bear dens', *Royal Society Open Science*, 2(4), 2015, 140022. http://doi.org/10.1098/rsos.140022

50 https://www.youtube.com/watch?v=zLSaDVG4yBE — retrieved 13/1/2024

51 Dassa, Ayelet, and Amir Dorit. 'The Role of Singing Familiar Songs in Encouraging Conversation Among People with Middle to Late Stage Alzheimer's Disease', *Journal of Music Therapy*, 51(2), 2014, pp. 131–53. https://doi.org/10.1093/jmt/thu007

52 https://www.youtube.com/watch?v=ezTrI7_jluI — retrieved 13/1/2024

53 Lorenz, Ralph. 'Health Benefits of Singing: A Perspective from Traditional Chinese Medicine and Chi Kung', *The Phenomenon of Singing*, 9, 2014, pp. 154–66.

54 https://www.youtube.com/watch?v=OwkUloxIJes — retrieved 13/1/2024

55 https://www.newscientist.com/article/mg25433861-200-fascia-the-long-overlooked-tissue-that-shapes-your-health/ — retrieved 13/1/2024

56 Perry, G., V. Polito, W.F. Thompson. 'Rhythmic Chanting and Mystical States across Traditions', *Brain Sciences*, 11(1), 2021, p. 101. https://doi.org/10.3390/brainsci11010101

57 Malviya, Shikha, Pamela Meredith, Barbra Zupan, and Lachlan Kerley. 'Identifying alternative mental health interventions: a systematic review of randomized controlled trials of chanting and breathwork', *Journal of Spirituality in Mental Health*, 24(2), 2022, pp. 191–233. DOI: 10.1080/19349637.2021.2010631

Chapter Six: Art

1 Kopaczyk, J.M., J. Warguła, and T. Jelonek. 'The variability of terpenes in conifers under developmental and environmental stimuli', *Environmental and Experimental Botany*, 180, 2020, 104197.

2   https://theconversation.com/trees-are-made-of-human-breath-99368 — retrieved 11/7/2024
3   https://www.youtube.com/watch?v=8nWM8UUSAUA&list=PLbFBbBFQ5o8w4rqc5RM9VUJ-jqdXXxtVy — retrieved 19/6/2024
4   Kimmerle, H. 'The world of spirits and the respect for nature: towards a new appreciation of animism', *The Journal for Transdisciplinary Research in Southern Africa*, 2(2), 2006, a277.
5   Peterson, N. 'Is the Aboriginal landscape sentient? Animism, the new animism and the Warlpiri', *Oceania*, 81(2), 2011, pp. 167–79.
6   De Castro, E.V. 'Perspectivism and Multinaturalism in Indigenous America', in Alexandre Surallés and Pedro García Herrera, eds., *The Land Within: Indigenous territory and perception of the environment*, International Work Group for Indigenous Affairs, 2005, p. 36.
7   'Nature And Us: A History through Art', BBC. https://www.bbc.co.uk/iplayer/episode/m0010jn6/nature-and-us-a-history-through-art-series-1-episode-1 — retrieved 18/6/2024
8   https://www.youtube.com/watch?v=VNSuETcYINU — retrieved 10/7/2024
9   https://www.youtube.com/watch?v=GPbWJPsBPdA — retrieved 11/7/2024
10 Joordens, J., F. d'Errico, F. Wesselingh, et al. '*Homo erectus* at Trinil on Java used shells for tool production and engraving', *Nature*, 518, 2015, pp. 228–31. https://doi.org/10.1038/nature13962
11 https://www.newscientist.com/article/mg25934530-200-these-ancient-sand-drawings-could-be-a-fifth-type-of-palaeoart/ — retrieved 12/12/2023
12 Fuentes, Agustín, Marc Kissel, Penny Spikins, Keneiloe Molopyane, John Hawks, and Lee R. Berger. 'Burials and

engravings in a small-brained hominin, *Homo naledi*, from the late Pleistocene: contexts and evolutionary implications', *eLife*, 12, 2023, RP89125. https://doi.org/10.7554/eLife.89125.1

13 Henshilwood, C.S., F. d'Errico, K.L. van Niekerk, et al. 'An abstract drawing from the 73,000-year-old levels at Blombos Cave, South Africa', *Nature*, 562, 2018, pp. 115–18. https://doi.org/10.1038/s41586-018-0514-3

14 https://www.britishmuseum.org/blog/lion-man-ice-age-masterpiece — retrieved 19/6/2024

15 https://en.wikipedia.org/wiki/Bicha_of_Balazote — retrieved 19/6/2024

16 http://mifologia.osipova-pr.com/soderjanie/slavyane/alkonost — retrieved 19/6/2024

17 https://www.britannica.com/topic/Echidna-Greek-mythology — retrieved 19/6/2024

18 https://worldhistoryedu.com/anansi-the-trickster-spider-man-of-west-africa/ — retrieved 19/6/2024

19 https://www.newscientist.com/article/2438291-50000-year-old-picture-of-a-pig-is-the-oldest-known-narrative-art/ — retrieved 11/7/2024

20 https://en.wikipedia.org/wiki/Munch_Bunch — retrieved 10/7/2024

21 Haviland, Virginia. *The Talking Pot*. Little, Brown & Company, 1990.

22 https://www.youtube.com/watch?v=JI4VReh9TLk — retrieved 11/7/2024

23 https://www.laits.utexas.edu/sami/diehtu/giella/art/mysticism.htm — retrieved 11/7/2024

24 Roberts, Rosebud O., Ruth H. Cha, Michelle M. Mielke, Yonas E. Geda Bradley F. Boeve, Mary M. Machulda, David S. Knopman, and Ronald C. Petersen, 'Risk and protective

factors for cognitive impairment in persons aged 85 years and older', *Neurology*, 84(18), 2015, pp. 1854–61.
25 https://twinstrust.org/static/89af4d2a-49fe-4d23-bbcf8475f099762f/5cdfb852-318c-4eb8-955ef8f6b8f5d6c0/Key-stats-and-facts.pdf — retrieved 12/12/2023
26 Freud, S. *Civilization and Its Discontents*. Penguin, 2002.
27 Cameron, Julia. *The Artist's Way*, Pan Macmillan, 1992.
28 https://theconversation.com/why-psychology-lost-its-soul-everything-comes-from-the-brain-54828 — retrieved 15/7/2024
29 https://indiginews.com/vancouver-island/healing-trauma-through-culture — retrieved 13/1/2022
30 https://www.nytimes.com/2018/06/07/well/how-i-used-art-to-get-through-trauma.html — retrieved 13/12/2023
31 https://static01.nyt.com/images/2018/05/17/well/00wellart-trauma1/00wellart-trauma1-superJumbo.jpg?quality=75&auto=webp — retrieved 13/12/2023
32 Junge, M.B. 'History of art therapy', in: D.E. Gussak and M.L. Rosal, eds., *The Wiley Handbook of Art Therapy*, Wiley Blackwell, 2016, pp. 7–16.
33 https://www.americanscientist.org/article/how-art-can-heal — retrieved 13/12/2023
34 Named after Douglas Adams, the science-fiction writer who suggested in his bestselling work, *The Hitchhiker's Guide to the Galaxy*, that 42 was the meaning of life.
35 https://en.wikipedia.org/wiki/Laschamp_event — retrieved 13/12/2023
36 https://theconversation.com/earths-magnetic-field-broke-down-42-000-years-ago-and-caused-massive-sudden-climate-change-155580 — retrieved 13/12/2023
37 Jöris, O., M. Street, T. Terberger, and B. Weninger. 'Radiocarbon Dating the Middle to Upper Palaeolithic

Transition: The Demise of the Last Neanderthals and the First Appearance of Anatomically Modern Humans in Europe', in: S. Condemi and G.C. Weniger, eds., *Continuity and Discontinuity in the Peopling of Europe. Vertebrate Paleobiology and Paleoanthropology*, Springer, 2011. https://doi.org/10.1007/978-94-007-0492-3_22

38 Cooper, Alan, et al., 'A global environmental crisis 42,000 years ago', *Science*, 371, 2021, pp. 811–18. DOI: 10.1126/science.abb8677

39 Mugerwa, S., and J.D. Holden. 'Writing therapy: a new tool for general practice?', *British Journal of General Practice*, 62(605), 2012, pp. 661–663. https://doi.org/10.3399/bjgp12X659457

40 McGuire, K.M., M.A. Greenberg, and R. Gevirtz. 'Autonomic effects of expressive writing in individuals with elevated blood pressure', *Journal of Health Psychology*, 10(2), 2005, pp. 197–209.

41 Lumley, M.A., J.C. Leisen, R.T. Partridge, et al. 'Does emotional disclosure about stress improve health in rheumatoid arthritis? Randomized, controlled trials of written and spoken disclosure', *Pain*, 152(4), 2011, pp. 866–77.

42 Van der Oord, S., S. Lucassen, AA. van Emmerik, and P.M. Emmelkamp. 'Treatment of post-traumatic stress disorder in children using cognitive behavioural writing therapy', *Clinical Psychology & Psychotherapy*, 17(3), 2010, pp. 240–9.

43 https://www.arts.gov/sites/default/files/US_Patterns_of_Arts_ParticipationRevised.pdf — retrieved 13/12/2023

44 https://www.gov.uk/government/statistics/taking-part-201920-arts/arts-taking-part-survey-201920 — retrieved 13/12/2023

45 https://www.un.org/en/desa/world-population-projected-reach-98-billion-2050-and-112-billion-2100 — retrieved 21/6/2024

46 https://www.un.org/development/desa/en/news/population/

our-world-is-growing-older.html — retrieved 21/6/2024
47 https://cks.nice.org.uk/topics/dementia/background-information/prevalence/ — retrieved 15/7/2024
48 https://bricksbristol.org/2024/04/welcome-building-public-art-programme-public-workshops-are-a-go/ — 15/7/2024
49 Guarnera, J., E. Yuen, and H. Macpherson. 'The Impact of Loneliness and Social Isolation on Cognitive Aging: A Narrative Review', *Journal of Alzheimer's Disease Reports*, 7(1), 2023, pp. 699–714. https://doi.org/10.3233/ADR-230011
50 https://www.youtube.com/watch?v=9mLd04uMJUU — retrieved 21/6/2024

Chapter Seven: Sleep

1 https://www.theguardian.com/lifeandstyle/2019/feb/08/how-modern-life-gets-in-the-way-of-sleep-chronic-insomnia — retrieved 14/9/2021
2 Samson, D.R., A.N. Crittenden, I.A. Mabulla, A.Z. Mabulla, and C.L. Nunn. 'Hadza sleep biology: Evidence for flexible sleep-wake patterns in hunter-gatherers', *American Journal of Physical Anthropology*, 162(3), 2017, pp. 573–82. DOI: 10.1002/ajpa.23160.
3 Wehr, Thomas A. 'In short photoperiods, human sleep is biphasic', *Journal of Sleep Research*, 1(2), 1992, pp. 103–7.
4 https://www.sleep.org/napping-around-the-world/ — retrieved 14/9/2021
5 Jung, Christopher, et al. 'Acute effects of bright light exposure on cortisol levels', *Journal of Biological Rhythms*, 25(3), 2010, pp. 208–16.
6 https://e360.yale.edu/digest/u-s-study-shows-widening-disconnect-with-nature-and-potential-solutions — retrieved 9/9/2021

7. https://news.mit.edu/2012/understanding-how-brains-control-our-habits-1029 — retrieved 15/9/2021
8. https://www.youtube.com/watch?v=_1V0rDSTC9I — retrieved 15/9/2021
9. Esaki, Y., K. Obayashi, K. Saeki, K Fujita, N. Iwata & T. Kitajima. 'Effect of nighttime bedroom light exposure on mood episode relapses in bipolar disorder'. *Acta psychiatrica Scandinavica*, 146(1), 2022, 64–73. https://doi.org/10.1111/acps.13422
10. https://academic.oup.com/sleep/article/42/4/zsz015/5289255 — retrieved 9/9/2021
11. Robb, A. *Why We Dream*. Houghton Mifflin Harcourt, 2018.
12. https://en.wikipedia.org/wiki/Jabberwocky#cite_note-Parsons-17 — retrieved 9/12/2023
13. https://www.bartleby.com/essay/Stephen-King-s-Insight-On-Dreams-PKQ3KJWKVU5YW — retrieved 11/12/2023
14. https://www.independent.co.uk/life-style/women/mary-shelley-movie-frankenstein-books-husband-trailer-biography-quotes-a8433531.html — retrieved 9/12/2023
15. Greene, Graham. *A World of My Own: a dream diary*. Open Road Integrated Media, Inc., 2018.
16. https://www.youtube.com/watch?v=lyu7v7nWzf0 — retrieved 11/1/2024
17. https://www.youtube.com/watch?v=PyHSu-trNt0 — retrieved 11/1/2024
18. https://www.classical5element.com/your-first-visit — retrieved 17/6/2024
19. Adams, J., C. Garcia, and G. Garg, 'Mugwort (*Artemisia vulgaris, Artemisia douglasiana, Artemisia argyi*) in the Treatment of Menopause, Premenstrual Syndrome, Dysmenorrhea and Attention Deficit Hyperactivity Disorder', *Chinese Medicine*,

3(3), 2012, pp. 116–23. DOI: 10.4236/cm.2012.33019.
20 Malinowski, Josie. *The Psychology of Dreaming*. Routledge, 2020.
21 Ekiert, H., J. Pajor, P. Klin, A. Rzepiela, H. Ślesak, and A. Szopa. 'Significance of *Artemisia Vulgaris* L. (Common Mugwort) in the History of Medicine and Its Possible Contemporary Applications Substantiated by Phytochemical and Pharmacological Studies', *Molecules*, 25(19), 2020, 4415. https://doi.org/10.3390/molecules25194415
22 https://herbalsupplements.health/plant/mugwort — retrieved 11/12/2023
23 https://www.youtube.com/watch?v=8NoeK5H4ZGw — retrieved 11/12/2023
24 https://www.youtube.com/watch?v=6Lwhyq45Fjk — retrieved 22/12/2023
25 https://www.youtube.com/watch?v=rZGalPW34Ig — retrieved 22/12/2023
26 *The Holy Bible, New International Version®, NIV®* Copyright © 1973, 1978, 1984, 2011 by Biblica, Inc.™ Used by permission. All rights reserved worldwide.
27 Höld, K.M., N.S. Sirisoma, T. Ikeda, T. Narahashi, and J.E. Casida. 'α-Thujone (the active component of absinthe): γ-Aminobutyric acid type A receptor modulation and metabolic detoxification', *Applied Biological Sciences*, 97(8), 2000, pp. 3826–31.
28 Margaria, R. 'Acute and sub-acute toxicity study on thujone', unpublished report of the Istituto di Fisiologia, Università di Milano, 1963 (cited from CoE Datasheet RD4. 2/14-44, 1999).
29 https://www.newscientist.com/article/mg24833073-600-how-the-strangeness-of-our-dreams-reveals-their-true-purpose/ — retrieved 11/12/2023

Chapter Eight: Death

1. https://link.springer.com/referenceworkentry/10.1007/978-3-030-24348-7_63 — retrieved 31/12/2023
2. https://www.newscientist.com/article/2230459-goop-lab-on-netflix-shows-how-easy-it-is-to-fall-for-bad-science/ — retrieved 13/1/2024
3. Savani, K., S. Kumar, N.V. Naidu, and C.S. Dweck. 'Beliefs about emotional residue: the idea that emotions leave a trace in the physical environment', *Journal of Personality and Social Psychology*, 101(4), 2011, pp. 684–701. https://doi.org/10.1037/a0024102
4. https://www.scientificamerican.com/article/believing-in-bad-vibes/ — retrieved 11/9/2023
5. Biabanaki, S.M. 'A Critical Analysis of Cognitive Explanations of Afterlife Belief', *Cumhuriyet İlahiyat Dergisi*, 24(2), 2020, pp. 749–64.
6. https://www.youtube.com/watch?v=hZB6RwJVHPc — retrieved 11/9/2023
7. https://www.youtube.com/watch?v=hZB6RwJVHPc — retrieved 11/9/2023
8. https://www.nature.com/scitable/topicpage/rosalind-franklin-a-crucial-contribution-6538012/ — retrieved 11/1/2024
9. Crick, Francis. *The Astonishing Hypothesis: The Scientific Search for the Soul*, Simon & Schuster, 1994. p. 3.
10. Bering, J. 'Intuitive Conceptions of Dead Agents' Minds: The Natural Foundations of Afterlife Beliefs as Phenomenological Boundary', *Journal of Cognition and Culture*, 2(4), 2002, pp. 263–308. https://doi.org/10.1163/15685370260441008
11. https://www.rep.routledge.com/articles/thematic/death/v-1/sections/the-mystery-of-death — retrieved 15/9/2023

12 https://www.theguardian.com/commentisfree/2021/aug/20/end-of-life-care-painful-death — retrieved 29/12/2023
13 https://nfda.org/news/statistics — retrieved 15/9/2023
14 https://en.wikipedia.org/wiki/List_of_countries_by_cremation_rate — retrieved 15/9/2023
15 https://www.nytimes.com/2020/12/14/travel/torajan-death-rituals-indonesia.html — retrieved 29/12/2023
16 https://www.theguardian.com/science/2015/sep/16/seroxat-study-harmful-effects-young-people — retrieved 31/12/2023
17 Medawar, Charles, and Andrew Herxheimer. 'A Comparison of Adverse Drug Reaction Reports from Professionals and Users, Relating to Risk of Dependence and Suicidal Behaviour with Paroxetine', *The International Journal of Risk and Safety in Medicine*, 16, 2004, pp. 5–19.
18 https://griefguide.sueryder.org/support/how-do-men-grieve/ — retrieved 31/12/2023
19 https://www.wellandgood.com/scheduling-grief/ — retrieved 30/12/2023
20 Monsó, S., and A.J. Osuna-Mascaró. 'Death is common, so is understanding it: the concept of death in other species', *Synthese*, 199(1-2), 2021, pp. 2251–75. https://doi.org/10.1007/s11229-020-02882-y
21 Dor-Ziderman, Y., Lutz, A., and A. Goldstein. 'Prediction-based neural mechanisms for shielding the self from existential threat', *NeuroImage*, 202, 2019, 116080. ISSN 1053-8119.
22 https://www.newscientist.com/article/mg26334992-900-why-taking-our-grief-out-into-nature-can-help-us-heal/ — retrieved 13/7/2024
23 Gyimes, I.L., and E. Valentini. 'Reminders of Mortality: Investigating the Effects of Different Mortality Saliences on Somatosensory Neural Activity', *Brain Sciences*, 13(7), 2023, 1077.

https://doi.org/10.3390/brainsci13071077

24 Bryant-Davis, T., and E.C. Wong. 'Faith to move mountains: Religious coping, spirituality, and interpersonal trauma recovery', *American Psychologist*, 68(8), 2013, pp. 675–84. https://doi.org/10.1037/a0034380

25 Kalish, Richard A. *The Final Transition*. Routledge, 1985.

26 Toh, W.L., N. Thomas, and S.L. Rossell. 'Auditory verbal hallucinations in bipolar disorder (BD) and major depressive disorder (MDD): A systematic review', *Journal of Affective Disorders*, 184, 2015, pp. 18–28. https://doi.org/10.1016/j.jad.2015.05.040